W9-AZM-126

Medicaid since 1980

Costs, Coverage, and the Shifting Alliance between the Federal Government and the States

THE URBAN INSTITUTE PRESS
Washington, D.C.

THE URBAN INSTITUTE PRESS
2100 M Street, N.W.
Washington, D.C. 20037

Library of Congress Cataloging in Publication Data

Medicaid since 1980: Costs, Coverage, and the Shifting Alliance between the Federal Government and the States / Teresa A. Coughlin, Leighton Ku, and John Holahan.

1. Medicaid.   I. Ku, Leighton.   II. Holahan, John.   III. Title.

HD7102.U4C638   1994   93-41868
368.4′2′00973—dc20   CIP

ISBN 0-87766-618-0 (paper, alk. paper)
ISBN 0-87766-617-2 (cloth, alk. paper)

Printed in the United States of America

Distributed by University Press of America
4720 Boston Way   3 Henrietta Street
Lanham, MD 20706   London WC2E 8LU ENGLAND

THE URBAN INSTITUTE is a nonprofit policy research and educational organization established in Washington, D.C., in 1968. Its staff investigates the social and economic problems confronting the nation and public and private means to alleviate them. The Institute disseminates significant findings of its research through the publications program of its Press. The goals of the Institute are to sharpen thinking about societal problems and efforts to solve them, improve government decisions and performance, and increase citizen awareness of important policy choices.

Through work that ranges from broad conceptual studies to administrative and technical assistance, Institute researchers contribute to the stock of knowledge available to guide decision making in the public interest.

Conclusions or opinions expressed in Institute publications are those of the authors and do not necessarily reflect the views of staff members, officers or trustees of the Institute, advisory groups, or any organizations that provide financial support to the Institute.

ACKNOWLEDGMENTS

This book would not have been possible without the support of our colleagues at the Urban Institute. David Heslam and David Liska worked tirelessly in editing and analyzing most of the Medicaid data presented in this report. Stephen Zuckerman helped develop the analytical framework for the decomposition of Medicaid growth. Korbin Liu provided numerous helpful suggestions for improving the report. Steven Puller and Lynn Tsoflias also provided invaluable assistance in many of the analyses. Joan Sanders skillfully oversaw the formating and word processing of the report.

Valuable help was also provided by colleagues outside the Institute. John Klemm and his associates at the Health Care Financing Administration made the Medicaid data available and also answered our questions; the analyses in this book could not have been conducted without their aid. Joshua Wiener of the Brookings Institution and James Tallon of the United Hospital Fund and the Kaiser Commission on the Future of Medicaid reviewed the manuscript and offered constructive suggestions and support. The Robert Wood Johnson Foundation and the Henry J. Kaiser Family Foundation generously provided funding for this work.

The opinions expressed in this book are the authors' and should not be interpreted as those of the Urban Institute or the two foundations.

CONTENTS

Tables

Figures

FOREWORD

Studying the U.S. health care system and alternative strategies to improve access and control costs has been central to the Urban Institute's mandate for the past two decades. Medicaid, the federal-state program implemented in the late 1960s to provide health care coverage for low-income Americans, has grown steadily throughout that period. Its budget is now well over $100 billion a year. It covers more than 35 million people. And it is the fastest growing item in most state budgets.

This volume is the third Urban Institute evaluation of the Medicaid program. Previous ones were completed in 1986 and 1990. Why do we need another study of Medicaid now, except for pure historical interest, at a time when health system reform may phase it out of existence?

The obvious answer is that what form health system reform will actually take is far from clear. Although some legislative proposals would replace Medicaid, the end result could include little more than tinkering. In that case, a comprehensive up-to-date analysis of Medicaid will be extremely important in guiding program reform.

But there is a more fundamental answer than that. Whether or not Medicaid continues, the problems with which it is contending will remain. Medicaid has grown from a program that served largely female-headed families on welfare to one that encompasses the whole range of health sector problems from infant mortality, to chronic disability, to nursing home care for the elderly. In trying to deal with the wide variety of problems that states are now including under their Medicaid umbrellas, Medicaid expenditures grew by over 28 percent from 1991 to 1992, in contrast to Medicare growth of under 11 percent and private insurance growth of under 8 percent over the same period. Understanding the reasons behind this explosive growth is crucial for any health care reform effort to be successful.

One major factor driving the growth was an intentional shifting of state-funded programs into Medicaid (to increase the federal matching funds available) and special state-developed financing programs that increase the federal match even more. These efforts are part of a broader pattern of tensions between state and federal governments over the Medicaid program, which has now become a major fiscal battleground in the struggle between governments. A sound understanding of the evolution of this battle is crucial to health reform efforts. Any new system, whatever its shape, will face the very problems states are now trying to solve with their Medicaid programs. Moreover, the history and legacy of Medicaid will shape the thinking and the response of state governments to any new intergovernmental health care partnership.

A final reason for this book is that many states have restructured their Medicaid programs over the past decade in ways that provide valuable experience from which national health system reform efforts can learn. This volume encapsulates the lessons learned from this experience, and uses them to examine how the current responsibilities of the Medicaid program might be configured under a variety of state and national reform proposals. The structure and financing of health care for low-income, disabled, and frail elderly Americans will remain a major focus of public policy, whatever the outcome of the current health care reform debate.

The Institute has been deeply engaged in providing technical and financial data to those in and out of government working on reform proposals. We hope and expect that this analysis will complement that assistance.

William Gorham
President

Chapter One

THE EVOLUTION OF MEDICAID 1981–92: AN OVERVIEW

The 1980s and early 1990s witnessed tremendous growth in the importance and visibility of Medicaid, the federal-state health insurance program for the poor, disabled, and medically needy. In 1981, Medicaid was a $28 billion program that served largely a cash welfare population. By 1992, it was a $113 billion program that enrolled more than 35 million people with diverse health, social, and insurance needs.

As Medicaid has grown, its mission has broadened and become increasingly complex. Today, the program struggles to deal with a wide variety of problems, ranging from the uninsured to long-term care to infant mortality. While these social problems exert intense pressure for continued program expansion, concern about escalating costs for Medicaid and the size of state and federal budgets demand that program growth be controlled. Indeed, Medicaid is now the fastest growing item in most state budgets. In 1992, Medicaid consumed about 5 percent of total federal spending, nearly double the percentage spent on the program in 1982.

This volume reviews and highlights the evolution of the Medicaid program between 1981 and 1992. (For readers less familiar with Medicaid, appendix 1.A provides a thumbnail sketch of the program.) With a special focus on the latter years, we use program data to evaluate Medicaid spending and enrollment trends over this period, in addition to documenting and discussing the many legislative changes that have occurred. This is the third such evaluation of the Medicaid program conducted by the Urban Institute; prior volumes have examined the program at earlier points in time (Holahan and Cohen 1986; Chang and Holahan 1990).

THE LAST DECADE AND MEDICAID

The years 1981 to 1992 brought significant changes to the Medicaid program. The early eighties saw a period of program retrenchment, largely as a consequence of the Omnibus Budget Reconciliation Act of 1981 (henceforth, OBRA 81). Passed in response to both rapidly accelerating Medicaid costs and pressure from the new Reagan administration, OBRA 81 made several major changes to Medicaid: it imposed a three-year reduction in the federal match of state expenditures and also reduced eligibility for welfare benefits, the latter being the usual entrée into the Medicaid program for poor families. In exchange for these reductions, states' options in delivering and paying for care were greatly broadened. It was during the early 1980s that states adopted new hospital payment systems and introduced alternative delivery systems such as health maintenance organizations (HMOs). Also during this period, states began to actively manage costs and services rather than simply pay bills.

Then, in the mid-1980s, the Medicaid program began a period of gradual expansion that continued through the end of the decade. As the economy improved, and as concern grew among federal and state policymakers that the OBRA 81 cutbacks were too severe, Congress enacted a series of laws requiring states to expand their programs. Between 1984 and 1990, Congress passed at least one major piece of legislation each year expanding Medicaid eligibility or service coverage. Many of these new laws were targeted to children and pregnant women. The rest of the expansions were directed to elderly and disabled persons and to other groups such as the homeless and newly legalized aliens. As part of these legislative changes, Medicaid's strong ties to the cash welfare system were greatly weakened, though not broken. These policy actions also substantially broadened the role of Medicaid in serving as the health care program for low-income persons.

In addition to the many federally legislated changes, program enrollment grew immensely during this period, rising from 25 million to over 35 million between 1984 and 1992. By 1992, nearly 1 in 7 Americans was enrolled in Medicaid, up from 1 in 10 in 1984.[1]

As Medicaid expanded to serve more people over the decade, program costs grew at an alarming rate—even when controlling for the increased enrollment. From 1981 to 1992, spending for Medicaid increased more than fourfold, expanding from $27.7 billion to $112.9 billion (figure 1.1). Growth, though, was highly uneven over the period. Throughout most of the early part of the 1980s, spending for Medicaid increased at or below 10 percent per year, slightly lower than the growth rates for Medicare and private health insurance. Then, beginning in the latter part of the decade, expenditure growth was particularly steep, increasing 13 percent in 1989, 19 percent in

Figure 1.1 MEDICAID EXPENDITURES, ENROLLEES, AND RATES OF GROWTH: 1981–92

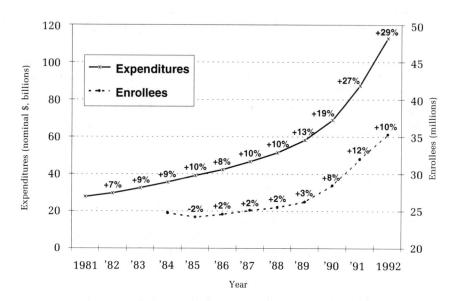

1990, 27 percent in 1991, and 29 percent in 1992. Even in inflation-adjusted dollars, recent spending increases have been dramatic. From 1989 to 1992, for example, average annual growth in constant dollars was 19 percent. These increases are the largest since Medicaid was established in 1965. In addition, when recent Medicaid expenditure patterns are compared to those of other major health insurors—Medicare and private health insurance—Medicaid's are dramatically different. Between 1990 and 1991, for example, Medicaid spending grew 28.1 percent per year. By contrast, over the same period, average annual growth rates for Medicare and private insurance were, respectively, 10.7 percent and 7.2 percent (Congressional Budget Office 1992).

Several recent studies have investigated the reasons for the surge in expenditure growth since the late 1980s (Congressional Budget Office 1992a; Congressional Research Service 1992; Feder et al. 1992). While generally indicating no single cause for the rapid expenditure growth, these studies have implicated a range of factors, including the federal Medicaid mandates, medical price inflation, and the recession. Beyond these, it also seems that states have intentionally accelerated growth by shifting previously state-funded programs into Medicaid, the so-called Medicaid maximization strategy.

States also have intentionally accelerated growth by establishing special financing programs such as provider donation and tax programs. Although operating in a variety of ways, these programs generally share the following characteristics: a provider makes a donation or tax payment to the state government, which, after receiving the federal match, sends back a larger payment to the provider, either in the form of higher reimbursement rates or a hospital disproportionate-share payment. (Since 1986 federal law has allowed state Medicaid programs to make special payments that exceed Medicare levels to hospitals that serve a disproportionately high level of low-income patients such as Medicaid and charity care patients.) The Health Care Financing Administration (HCFA) has estimated that in fiscal year (FY) 1992 alone states collected about $8 billion from provider tax and donation programs and spent more than $16 billion in disproportionate-share payments. Some of the money generated from special revenue programs was used to cover Medicaid expenses, whereas some covered expenses completely outside of Medicaid. One consequence of special financing programs is that the programs have greatly distorted recent Medicaid spending trends, particularly state spending trends.

These state efforts to shift costs to the federal government are part of a broader pattern of tension between state and federal governments over Medicaid. Whereas states initially supported the Medicaid expansions for pregnant women and children, they became increasingly concerned about the costs associated with them and other federally mandated Medicaid expansions. Concern quickly escalated to alarm as states tried to implement the expansions while dealing with severe budget constraints caused by the recent recession. At the same time, states' use of programs such as provider taxes caused ire at the federal level, eventually resulting in passage of the 1991 Medicaid Voluntary Contributions and Provider-Specific Tax Amendments. This law sharply limited states' use of special financing programs. As Medicaid grew over the decade, the increasing fiscal burden of the program strained not only state and federal pocketbooks but intergovernmental relations as well. Preliminary data indicate that Medicaid growth in 1993 slowed substantially, largely due to the 1991 law capping these programs.

Although Medicaid has become a greater problem at state and federal levels, it has been overshadowed by much broader concerns about the medically uninsured and runaway health care costs in general. Within the past few years, virtually every state has considered or initiated health care reforms, many of which call for significant changes in the Medicaid program. Most recently, in September 1993 President Clinton unveiled a sweeping national health care reform proposal that would provide all Americans with access to health care while limiting growth of costs through managed competition and global budgets. The Clinton proposal would radically restructure Medicaid as we know it today: most acute and preventive care services for current Medicaid enrollees would be provided under the same regional health alliances that would provide care to privately insured persons. Long-term care (such as nursing home care and intermediate care facilities for the mentally retarded—ICFs/MR) and certain other services (such as dental and chiropractic services) would form the "residual" Medicaid program.

As of this writing, it is too early to predict the timing or course of health care system reform. In addition to the President's plan, a variety of other legislative proposals have been introduced, ranging from a voluntary individual mandate to a single public payor system. Thus precisely how the Medicaid program will be affected if health care reform is adopted is at present unclear. National health care reform may replace Medicaid altogether. Alternatively, small, incremental adjustments to Medicaid may be the result of the health reform discussions. Whatever lies ahead, though, it is important to evaluate the recent Medicaid experience. As outlined above, the program has undergone substantial changes since the late 1980s: Over the years, Medicaid's coverage of the population greatly expanded and program costs soared. In addition, Medicaid became a fiscal battleground between the federal and state governments as to how to divide program expenditures. A sound understanding of the evolution of these events would be most helpful in charting the future, particularly if major restructuring is contemplated.

ORGANIZATION OF THIS VOLUME

Chapter 2 of this volume describes broad expenditure and enrollment trends between 1981 and 1992, with a special focus on the years 1988–92. The following issues are examined:

□ Why has federal expenditure growth outpaced state expenditure growth?
□ What factors have contributed to the rapid expenditure growth since the late 1980s? Is this acceleration likely to continue?

▢ How does growth in Medicaid expenditures compare to growth in other insurance markets such as Medicare and private health? Is Medicaid expenditure growth really out of control?
▢ Where has the expenditure growth been concentrated: in long-term care services or acute care services?

Chapter 3 discusses trends in Medicaid eligibility policy between 1981 and 1991. We evaluate how these patterns affected Medicaid enrollment for various groups and how they relate to overall poverty and medical insurance trends during the decade. Specifically, the chapter addresses the following questions:

▢ How has the composition of the Medicaid population changed? Have some groups grown faster than others?
▢ Has variation among the states for eligibility changed during the decade?
▢ What has been the impact of the federal mandates on program enrollment?
▢ Did the broadening of eligibility policies improve coverage of the poor? Did it improve coverage of the uninsured?

Throughout the 1980s, a variety of changes aimed at reducing Medicaid program inequities among the states were implemented. Such changes include the federal mandates, "bootstrap" financing, and Boren Amendment lawsuits. Chapter 4 evaluates whether states' Medicaid programs became more comparable over the 1980s. In particular, the following questions are considered:

▢ Has program coverage become more equitable nationwide?
▢ Have expenditures per recipient become more similar across the states?

Chapter 5 examines how the recent Medicaid expenditure growth was financed by states. Specifically, the following questions are discussed:

▢ How did states pay for Medicaid expenditure growth?
▢ What was the role of special financing programs such as provider tax and donation programs?

Chapters 6 and 7 review changing expenditures and policies at the level of specific services. Chapter 6 addresses long-term care services, while chapter 7 addresses acute and preventive care services. In particular, we consider the following issues:

□ What have been the broad spending trends for each of the major services since the mid-1980s?
□ What explains the differing growth rates: changes in policy, enrollment, or payment rates?
□ How have acute care services fared relative to long-term care services?

We conclude in chapter 8 with a discussion of this volume's major findings. We also highlight some of the many state efforts to restructure their Medicaid programs and briefly examine how the Medicaid program might be configured under a variety of state and national health care reform proposals.

Note

1. *Enrollment* refers to those individuals who were enrolled in Medicaid at any point during a given year. Program enrollment is distinct from program recipients (an often-used measure of program size) in that enrollees do not necessarily receive services whereas all recipients do. The data used in this report to estimate program enrollment and other statistics are discussed in full in chapter 2.

WHAT IS MEDICAID? A BRIEF GUIDE

Enacted in 1965 as a companion to Medicare, Medicaid is a federal safety net program that pays for medical and long-term care for those who cannot afford care owing to poverty, old age, or physical or mental disability. Medicaid is a means-tested entitlement program that is financed jointly by federal and state governments. Eligible people are legally entitled to receive services, and providers are legally entitled to be reimbursed. There are no program caps on expenditure levels.

Although financed jointly, Medicaid is administered by the states and the District of Columbia within broad federal guidelines. Because of this design feature, each state determines whom and what to cover and how much providers will be paid. Thus, Medicaid is, in reality, a compilation of 51 uniquely different programs, making it probably the most complex of the nation's social assistance programs. Here we summarize only the key aspects of Medicaid. Since states are allowed considerable discretion in program structure, there is no standard set of program rules. The policies summarized here thus have many exceptions. (For a comprehensive reference, see Congressional Research Service 1993.)

Who Can Participate?   Under Medicaid law, states are required to cover some groups, whereas others are optional. In the following listing of main groups, the first three are mandatory and the remaining two are optional.

1. *Persons receiving AFDC or SSI.* All recipients of Aid to Families with Dependent Children (AFDC) or Supplemental Security Income (SSI) are usually covered. The AFDC program covers poor single-parent families and two-parent families with an unemployed principal earner, whereas the SSI program covers poor, blind, and disabled persons. Combined, AFDC and SSI recipients account for the bulk of Medicaid enrollees.

2. *Low-income children and pregnant women.* Through a series of federal mandates passed in the 1980s, Medicaid coverage has recently been extended to low-income children and pregnant women whose income exceeds AFDC financial eligibility standards.
3. *Low-income Medicare beneficiaries.* Included in the 1988 Medicare Catastrophic Cost Act (MCAA), Medicaid is now required to pay Medicare premiums, deductibles, and coinsurance for low-income aged and disabled Medicare beneficiaries. This group is referred to as the qualified Medicare beneficiaries or "QMBs."
4. *The medically needy.* States have the option to provide coverage to individuals who meet the program's categorical standards (for example, they are aged, blind, disabled, pregnant, or a child) but whose incomes are higher than allowed by the program. Such individuals can be entitled to coverage because their medical bills are so high that they deplete their income and assets to some predetermined level. This process of asset and income depletion is often referred to as spenddown. While all services can be provided under this option, most medically needy expenditures cover long-term care services, particularly for the elderly.
5. *Persons requiring institutional care.* States also have the option to provide long-term care to categorically eligible individuals whose incomes exceed program standards and who are receiving care in nursing facilities or intermediate care facilities for the mentally retarded (ICFs/MR). Under Medicaid law, states can cover such individuals whose incomes are up to 300 percent of the SSI limit.

What Health Services Do Clients Get?   To earn federal financing help, states are required to provide a basic set of services. States are also allowed to provide several optional services.

☐ *Mandatory Services that States Must Offer:* Hospital care (inpatient and outpatient); physician services; nursing home services, home health services, laboratory and X-ray services; Medicare premiums, deductibles, and copayments; preventive health services for children; family planning; clinic services.
☐ *Optional Services that States May Offer:* Prescription drugs, intermediate care facilities for the mentally retarded, inpatient mental health for children and elderly, personal care, and other health services such as dental, optometric, podiatric, chiropractic, and transportation services.

Typically services are rendered free of charge to recipients. Medicaid beneficiaries can obtain care from any participating physician, hospital, or other health care provider. A persistent problem in the program, however, is that many providers, particularly physicians, have chosen not to participate largely because Medicaid reimbursement rates tend to be low relative to the private sector and Medicare. Thus, access to providers is often difficult for Medicaid recipients. To counteract this problem, in an increasing number of states, Medicaid beneficiaries may join, or may even be required to join, managed care plans. While this shift may improve access, it restricts, beneficiaries' choice of health care providers. Some Medicaid beneficiaries also have other insurance, such as Medicare or private health insurance. In these cases, Medicaid supplements the other insurance as a payer of last resort.

Who Pays for Medicaid?   As mentioned earlier, Medicaid is a federal-state partnership in which both levels of government share program costs. The federal government pays for 50 percent to 80 percent of total Medicaid costs. The federal matching percentage is determined by a formula based on the per capita income of each state; poorer states get more federal matching. A controversial innovation is that many states have recently developed special financing programs in which provider taxes, provider donations, or intergovernmental transfers have been used to leverage higher federal matching payments.

Who Administers Medicaid?   At the federal level, Medicaid is administered by the Health Care Financing Administration (HCFA), which is part of the U.S. Department of Health and Human Services (DHHS). At the state level, the administering agencies vary and include state health or human service departments.

Chapter Two

MEDICAID SPENDING AND ENROLLMENT TRENDS, 1981–92

Total federal and state expenditures for Medicaid spiraled from almost $28 billion in 1981 to nearly $113 billion in 1992, an average annual growth rate of 13.6 percent. Growth has been particularly rapid in the last few years: since 1988, spending has more than doubled. Partly mirroring the increases in expenditures, program enrollment has also swelled. Between 1984 and 1992, the number of persons enrolled in Medicaid increased by more than 10 million, with much of the growth occurring since 1988.

This chapter examines overall Medicaid expenditure and enrollment patterns since 1981. We begin with a brief discussion of the data sources and methods used to conduct this examination. Then we look at total spending both by type of payer (federal or state) and broad service category (acute care or long-term care). We then examine spending, as well as program enrollment trends, by eligibility group. We conclude with an investigation of the principal factors that have contributed to the recent surge in program expenditures.

DATA SOURCES AND METHODS

Data Sources

Most of the Medicaid expenditure and enrollment data used in this book are based on state Medicaid reports submitted to the Health Care Financing Administration (HCFA), the federal agency responsible for the overall management of the Medicaid program. Specifically, data were taken from the HCFA-2082 and the HCFA-64 reporting forms. Each of these reports has strengths and weaknesses. HCFA-2082 is an annual statistical report about Medicaid recipients and enrollment, with detailed listings by eligibility category. It also contains expenditure data, but these are sometimes unreliable (Ku, Ellwood, and Klemm 1990). HCFA-64, by contrast, is a quarterly budget report that states submit to receive federal matching dollars. It contains the most accurate Medicaid financial data. The disadvantage of the HCFA-64 is that it has relatively little data on recipient characteristics.

Drawing on the strengths of each report, we created a merged dataset using expenditure data from the HCFA-64 and enrollment and recipiency data from the HCFA-2082. Once combined, the dataset was edited and cleaned to reconcile inconsistencies or gaps. Since the HCFA-2082 reports do not include information about HMO/group health or Medicare payments, there are no corresponding enrollment or recipiency data available for these services. Thus, we used data from the HCFA-64 for these services. This merged dataset forms the basis for most of the analyses contained in this book. (Throughout the book, however, we do use a variety of other sources to supplement the HCFA Medicaid program data, including the Current Population Survey of the U.S. Bureau of the Census and data from the National Association of State Budget Officers. Supplemental data sources are described when introduced.)

Recipients versus Enrollees

In addition to creating a merged dataset, we also created a complete time-series of Medicaid program enrollment. The HCFA-2082 has historically collected information on the number of *recipients*, that is, persons who actually received one or more services. Only recently has the HCFA-2082 asked states to submit information on the number of *enrollees*, that is, persons enrolled in Medicaid regardless of whether they used a service. The distinction between recipients and enrollees is important: recipiency measures service use, whereas enrollment measures the total Medicaid population, both service users and nonusers.[1] Number of enrollees, thus, is a broader, more comprehensive measure of Medicaid coverage. For most of our analyses, we evaluated the Medicaid population in terms of enrollees rather than recipients. In some instances, however, recipients were used instead. In evaluating long-term care services, for example, it made better sense to analyze expenditures in terms of recipients rather than enrollees because relatively fewer people actually use such services.

As noted earlier, states' submission of enrollment data has only recently become mandatory, though many states have submitted it voluntarily for several years. To generate a time-series of enrollment for each state, we imputed missing enrollment data using reported recipient levels and the historical relationship between the number of recipients and enrollees.

Data Exclusions

The expenditure data presented here may differ from other reports because of two exclusions. We did not include administrative expenditures or accounting adjustments (which cannot be allocated to a specific service) for Medicaid; instead, our dataset includes only vendor payments (that is, payments made for health care.) Excluding administrative expenditures reduces spending by about 4 percent. Because of unique program features and federal matching arrangements, we also excluded data from Arizona and the U.S. territories (Puerto Rico, Virgin Islands, Guam, American Samoa, and the Northern Marianas).[2] In 1992, these exclusions amounted to about $3 billion.

Price Index

Much of our expenditure data are presented in real or constant dollars, rather than nominal dollars. The base year for our analysis was 1992. Selecting appropriate price inflation indexes for Medicaid is inherently difficult, since state Medicaid programs set many prices through their reimbursement mechanisms. The price index we employed, an updated version of one developed by Holahan and Cohen (1986), attempts to measure inflation for the health care sector as a composite of several services. The indexes do not measure actual Medicaid price changes; instead they price changes for the general health care system.

The Medicaid service-specific price indexes we constructed draw from two general price indexes—the Medical Care-Consumer Price Index (MC-CPI) and the HCFA market basket indexes. The MC-CPI indexes are based on consumer-level prices charged for services or goods provided by physicians, pharmacists, and so on. The HCFA market basket indexes are indicators of the prices of key inputs to services; for example, the salaries of doctors and nurses and cost of medical supplies and equipment. The specific components of the MC-CPI and the market basket used to create the Medicaid price index are described in more detail in appendix A.

MEDICAID EXPENDITURE TRENDS, 1981–92

Although expenditure growth for Medicaid averaged about 14 percent per year between 1981 and 1992, growth was highly uneven throughout the period (table 2.1). In the 1981–84 period, Medicaid spending increased at 8.6 percent per year in nominal dollars. After adjusting for price inflation, growth was only about 1 percent. This low growth rate occurred even though the nation was in a deep recession, which increased the rate of poverty. Most likely, the low rate reflects the impact of the cost-containment measures included in OBRA 81, which, among other things, gave states considerable latitude in designing lower-cost reimbursement and alternative delivery systems. The legislation also temporarily reduced the federal match rate and restricted welfare eligibility (Holahan and Cohen 1986).

From 1984 to 1987, the pace of spending quickened to around 10 percent per year (5 percent after adjusting for inflation) (table 2.1). This increased spending rate stems, in part, from the federal legislation passed in this period requiring states to expand Medicaid program eligibility and services, such as the pregnant women and children eligibility expansions and the Early Periodic Screening, Diagnostic, and Treatment (EPSDT) service expansions for children (Chang and Holahan 1990).

Beginning in 1989, Medicaid spending greatly accelerated. Total yearly nominal expenditures from 1989 to 1992 increased by 13 percent in 1989, 19 percent in 1990, 27 percent in 1991, and 29 percent in 1992 (table 2.1). Even in constant dollars, the expenditure surge has been dramatic, with constant dollar spending for Medicaid increasing by double digits each year since 1989. Preliminary data indicate Medicaid spending growth was 10 percent, substantially below the '91 and '92 growth levels.

The extraordinary growth that has occurred over the last few years is a departure from historic Medicaid spending trends. During most of the 1980s, Medicaid spending growth was comparable to that of the other major payers—private health insurance and Medicare (Congressional Budget Office 1992b). From 1983 to 1987, for example, the average annual expenditure growth rate was 9.9 percent for Medicaid, 7.9 percent for private health insurance, and 8.5 percent for Medicare (table 2.2). By contrast, between 1987 and 1990, the annual expenditure growth rate for Medicaid jumped to 13.7 percent, whereas growth rates for private insurance and Medicare were,

Table 2.1 MEDICAID EXPENDITURES BY SOURCE OF PAYMENT: 1981–92

Year(s)	Total		Federal		State/Local	
	Nominal ($ billions)	1992 Constant ($ billions)	Nominal ($ billions)	1992 Constant ($ billions)	Nominal ($ billions)	1992 Constant ($ billions)
1981	27.7	50.2	15.6	28.3	12.1	21.9
1984	35.4	52.0	19.5	28.7	15.9	23.3
1987	46.6	60.9	26.0	33.9	20.6	26.9
1988	51.3	63.7	28.7	35.7	22.6	28.0
1989	58.1	67.8	32.6	38.1	25.4	29.6
1990	69.0	75.8	38.9	42.8	30.1	33.0
1991	87.4	91.0	49.6	51.7	37.8	39.3
1992	112.9	112.9	64.7	64.7	48.2	48.2
Average Annual Percentage Change:						
1981–84	8.6%	1.2%	7.8%	0.5%	9.6%	2.1%
1984–87	9.5	5.4	10.0	5.8	9.0	4.9
1987–88	10.1	4.6	10.5	5.1	9.5	4.1
1988–89	13.2	6.4	13.8	6.9	12.6	5.8
1989–90	18.8	11.9	19.2	12.2	18.4	11.5
1990–91	26.7	20.1	27.5	20.9	25.6	19.1
1991–92	29.1	24.0	30.3	25.1	27.6	22.5
1981–92	13.6	7.6	13.8	7.8	13.4	7.4

Note: Arizona and U.S. territories are not included.

Table 2.2 NATIONAL HEALTH EXPENDITURES: AVERAGE ANNUAL GROWTH
RATES BY SOURCE OF FUNDS, 1983–1992

	Year		
	1983–1987	1987–1990	1990–1992
Average Annual Growth Rate	8.4%	10.4%	10.1%
Private	7.9	10.3	7.2
Government	9.2	10.5	14.1
Medicare	8.5	10.2	10.7
Medicaid	9.9	13.7	28.1
Other	9.6	8.6	6.1

Source: U.S. Congressional Budget Office, 1992.

respectively, 10.5 and 10.2. The expenditure growth rate for Medicaid
relative to private insurance and Medicare became even more disparate between 1990 and 1992.

Medicaid Spending and the Federal/State Partnership

Table 2.1 also shows how expenditures have been shared by Medicaid's two payers—the federal government and state and local governments—since 1981. Although overall spending growth rates for
both payers have been comparable, the relative rates have varied
from year to year. At the start of the decade, expenditure growth was
much greater for state and local governments than for the federal
government. This was largely a consequence of OBRA 81, which, as
mentioned earlier, temporarily reduced the federal match. By the
middle of the decade, however, federal expenditure growth began to
outpace state and local spending growth. This trend continued
through 1992.

A variety of factors contributed to the escalated growth in federal
Medicaid spending. In 1984, as federal spending started to grow
faster than state spending, the federal mandates requiring expansion
of Medicaid began to be implemented. The mandates most affected
the spending growth rates of southern states, which traditionally had
less-generous Medicaid programs. At the same time, southern states
have the highest federal Medicaid match rates. Thus, the southern
states' large growth rates, coupled with their high match rates, have
contributed to the disproportionate increase in the federal share of
Medicaid spending.

Another factor contributing to widening growth rates between federal and state spending is the states' increasing reliance on special

financing programs such as provider tax and donation programs. Since these programs have been used more extensively by southern states—which have the higher match rates—the effect on federal spending growth has been particularly large.

Overlaying the impact of the mandates and special financing mechanisms, structural changes in the federal match rate have also fueled the recent accelerated growth of federal spending. The federal match rate, formally known as the Federal Medicaid Assistance Percentage (FMAP), is based on a state's per capita personal income relative to the whole nation. It is annually updated to account for shifts in states' income. Throughout the 1980s states' relative incomes were redistributed in a manner that brought about an increase in the average FMAP. A by-product of this redistribution is that federal spending relative to state and local spending grew at a higher rate. One recent study estimated that had the 1986 FMAP been in place in 1992, the federal share of spending would have been $1.5 billion lower (Miller 1992).

Share of Medicaid Spending for Long-Term Care Is Diminishing

The recent escalation in program expenditures accompanies a diminishing dominance of long-term care in Medicaid. Table 2.3, which splits Medicaid expenditures (in constant 1992 dollars) since 1984 into three broad service categories—long-term care, hospital inpatient care, and all other acute care—illustrates that until most recently spending for long-term care was comparable to spending for hospital inpatient and other acute care combined. As late as 1987, for example, nearly half, 48 percent, of Medicaid expenditures went toward long-term care, 23 percent went toward inpatient care, and 29 percent went toward other acute care such as physician and hospital outpatient care. By 1992, spending for long-term care accounted for less than 40 percent of total program expenditures.

Much of the shift away from long-term care spending can be accounted for by the exceptionally high growth in inpatient hospital spending that began in 1990 and continued through 1992. Inpatient expenditures grew by 20 percent in 1990, 42 percent in 1991, and 41 percent in 1992. Moreover, hospital inpatient spending accounted for half of total Medicaid expenditure growth in both 1991 and 1992. By 1992, spending on hospital inpatient care alone surpassed spending for all other acute care services combined. These extremely rapid expenditure increases are a dramatic break from past hospital spending patterns. As recently as 1989, for example, the hospital expendi-

Table 2.3 MEDICAID EXPENDITURES BY BROAD SERVICE CATEGORY: 1984–92
(CONSTANT 1992 DOLLARS)

	1984	1985	1986	1987	1988	1989	1990	1991	1992
Expenditures (billions)									
Inpatient hospital	$12.8	$12.9	$13.4	$14.2	$14.5	$15.6	$18.7	$26.4	$37.2
Other acute care[a]	15.1	15.9	17.0	17.9	19.1	20.9	23.1	27.3	32.0
Long-term care[b]	24.2	26.3	27.0	28.7	30.1	31.3	34.1	37.3	43.6
Total	52.0	55.1	57.4	60.9	63.7	67.8	75.8	91.0	112.9
Growth Rates									
Inpatient hospital		0.7%	3.9%	6.0%	2.5%	7.1%	19.8%	41.6%	41.0%
Other acute care		5.9	6.9	5.2	6.4	9.4	10.5	18.5	17.2
Long-term care		8.6	2.8	6.5	4.6	4.1	8.9	9.5	17.0
Total		5.9	4.2	6.0	4.6	6.4	11.9	20.1	24.0
Share of Growth									
Inpatient hospital		2.8%	21.4%	23.4%	12.5%	25.4%	38.3%	50.9%	49.6%
Other acute care		29.1	47.1	25.9	40.4	44.1	27.2	27.9	21.5
Long-term care		68.1	31.4	50.7	47.1	30.5	34.5	21.2	29.0

Note: Arizona and U.S. territories are not included.

a. "Other acute care" represents the combined expenditures for physician/laboratory/X-ray, outpatient, prescription drugs, EPSDT, payments to Medicare, payments to HMOs, and expenditures for other specific services such as vision care, family planning, and dental care.

b. "Long-term care" represents the combined expenditures for SNF/ICF-other, ICF-MR, mental health, and home and community-based care.

ture growth rate was only 7.1 percent (table 2.3). Growth rates were lower still in earlier years. As discussed later in this and other chapters, recent hospital spending levels are greatly distorted by the states' use of special financing programs.

Although not as spectacular as inpatient expenditure growth, spending for other acute care has also greatly increased over the last several years. In fact, with the exception of the years 1987 and 1990–92, spending growth for other acute care outpaced spending increases for inpatient care since 1984 and, except for 1987, outpaced spending increases for long-term care since 1986 (table 2.3).

Finally, it is important to note the mounting growth in long-term care expenditures that occurred from 1990 to 1992. For reasons to be discussed in chapter 6, long-term care spending grew by 9 percent in 1990, 10 percent in 1991, and 17 percent in 1992 (table 2.3). These recent spending increases represent dramatic upward shifts in spending: from 1984 to 1989, annual increases for long-term care were about 5 percent (table 2.3).

Although in recent years acute care spending has overall increased at a faster rate than long-term care spending, the spending growth for acute care will likely subside as the use of special financing programs, such as provider tax and donation programs, diminishes. Long-term care, by contrast, will probably continue to be an important contributor to expenditure growth in the future.

Spending and Enrollment Trends across Eligibility Groups, 1981–92

While spending growth for acute and hospital inpatient services has greatly outpaced spending for long-term care services, the aged and the blind and disabled continue to consume the bulk of Medicaid expenditures. These two groups combined accounted for 67 percent of total expenditures in 1992, whereas adults and children accounted for 33 percent of expenditures (table 2.4). This expenditure balance between the long-term care populations and the acute care populations has been quite consistent: in 1981, for example, spending for the aged and blind and disabled accounted for 71 percent of expenditures, and spending for adults and children accounted for 29 percent.

Also stable has been the overall composition of the Medicaid population (table 2.5). Since 1984, the aged and the blind and disabled have accounted for about one-quarter of Medicaid enrollees (that is, the total number of persons enrolled in Medicaid, both users and nonusers), with adults and children accounting for the remainder.

Table 2.4 MEDICAID EXPENDITURES BY ELIGIBILITY GROUP: 1981–92
(CONSTANT 1992 DOLLARS)

Year(s)	Total ($ billions)[a]	Aged ($ billions)	Blind and Disabled ($ billions)	Adults ($ billions)	Children ($ billions)
1981	49.9	18.0	17.2	7.1	7.6
1984	50.4	18.9	17.7	6.8	7.0
1987	58.7	21.4	21.9	7.1	8.3
1988	61.2	22.1	23.2	7.3	8.7
1989	64.6	22.4	24.8	8.0	9.3
1990	72.5	24.3	27.5	9.5	11.2
1991	87.0	27.6	32.3	12.2	14.8
1992	108.0	32.2	39.9	15.5	20.4
Average Annual Percentage Change:					
1981–84	0.3%	1.7%	1.0%	−1.8%	−2.6%
1984–87	5.2	4.1	7.3	1.8	5.8
1987–88	4.2	3.3	6.0	1.8	4.0
1988–89	5.5	1.4	6.8	10.6	8.0
1989–90	12.3	8.5	11.0	18.3	19.7
1990–91	20.0	13.7	17.5	28.6	32.5
1991–92	24.1	16.8	23.4	26.4	37.6
1981–92	7.3	5.4	8.0	7.3	9.4

Note: Arizona and U.S. territories are not included.
a. Numbers do not sum to total amounts shown in table 2.1 because HMO payments and payments to Medicare are not included, since these cannot be distributed to specific eligibility groups because these payments are not reported on the HCFA-2082.

This is despite the exceptionally high enrollment increases for adults and children that began in 1989, following the passage of the federal mandates expanding Medicaid coverage of children and pregnant women.

Thus, even though the Medicaid population overwhelmingly comprises children and adults, the bulk of expenditures go toward care of the elderly and the blind and disabled. This seeming anomaly is the product of the significantly higher costs associated with caring for the latter groups. In 1992, for example, HCFA-64 and -2082 data indicated that the average spending per enrollee was $8,562 for aged persons and $8,268 for blind and disabled persons, respectively. By contrast, per enrollee spending for adults was $1,879; for children, the cost was $1,105. Most of the spending difference is attributed to the high use of institutional services, particularly long-term care services, by the elderly and the blind and disabled.

Although overall spending patterns and program composition

Table 2.5 NUMBER OF MEDICAID ENROLLEES BY ELIGIBILITY GROUP:
1984–92

Year(s)	Total (thousands)	Aged (thousands)	Blind and Disabled (thousands)	Adults (thousands)	Children (thousands)
1984	25,041	3,279	3,167	5,897	12,697
1987	25,249	3,207	3,507	5,874	12,662
1988	25,492	3,202	3,604	5,896	12,790
1989	26,236	3,286	3,791	6,073	13,086
1990	28,433	3,397	3,982	6,692	14,363
1991	31,967	3,571	4,327	7,560	16,509
1992	35,292	3,761	4,826	8,249	18,456
Average Annual Percentage Change:					
1984–87	0.3%	−0.7%	3.5%	−0.1%	−0.1%
1987–88	1.0	−0.1	2.8	0.4	1.0
1988–89	2.9	2.6	5.2	3.0	2.3
1989–90	8.4	3.4	5.0	10.2	9.8
1990–91	12.4	5.1	8.7	13.0	14.9
1991–92	10.4	5.3	11.5	9.1	11.8
1984–92	4.4	1.7	5.4	4.3	4.8

Note: Arizona and U.S. territories are not included.

between the aged and disabled and adults and children have remained stable, some important shifts across the individual categories have occurred. Most noteworthy is that the blind and disabled now represent the largest share of Medicaid expenditures: in 1992, Medicaid spent $40 billion caring for the blind and disabled, about 37 percent of total program expenditures. Although expenditures for the aged (at $32 billion) closely followed those for the blind and disabled, the aged had consistently dominated Medicaid spending until the late 1980s (see table 2.4).

The fact that spending for the blind and disabled has surpassed that for the aged can be attributed in part to disparate enrollment growth rates experienced by the two groups throughout the 1980s. Between 1984 and 1992, the blind and disabled were the single fastest growing eligibility group, increasing an average of 5.4 percent each year (table 2.5). By contrast, enrollment growth for the aged was the slowest over the period.

As discussed in chapter 3. a variety of factors have contributed to the rapid enrollment growth for the blind and disabled, including the recent 1990 Supreme Court decision in *Sullivan v. Zebley*, which required retroactive determination of eligibility to 1980 for disabled children (Sullivan v. Zebley, 1990). Another factor is that in recent years, proportionally more of the disabled are now covered by Supplemental Security Income (SSI)—automatically entitling them to Medicaid coverage. In addition, some have speculated that the recession may be a contributing factor, in that disabled persons often lose their jobs during economic downturns and, in turn, their employer-based health insurance coverage (Congressional Research Service 1992).

WHY ARE MEDICAID COSTS SKYROCKETING?

What specific factors brought about the rapid escalation in Medicaid spending? The federal mandates? Medical care price inflation? Increases in program enrollment? Increases in provider reimbursement? Moreover, to what extent has each of these factors contributed to the growth?

To investigate these issues, we developed a model that decomposes the relative roles of various factors we believe influenced the recent surge in Medicaid expenditures. Specifically, the model calculates how much each individual growth factor contributed to overall expenditure increases. The general model assumes that expenditure growth is the product of three factors: increases in the number of enrollees, medical price inflation, and increases in expenditures per enrollee over and above inflation. The share of total expenditure growth was calculated for each service type (inpatient hospital care, nursing home care, and the like) by each eligibility group (aged, children, adults, and blind and disabled). As noted earlier, the merged HCFA 64-2082 dataset did not allow us to separate Medicaid payments to Medicare and HMOs by eligibility groups; hence, these expenditure items were treated as separate growth factors. Appendix B describes the decomposition model in fuller detail.

Between 1988 and 1992, Medicaid expenditures grew from $51.3 billion to $112.9 billion, an increase of more than $61 billion (in nominal dollars) (table 2.1). In broad terms, of this $61 billion increase, the decomposition model estimated that 36 percent can be attributed to increases in the number of Medicaid recipients, 26 percent can be attributed to medical care price inflation, and 33 percent can be attributed to service use and reimbursement above inflation (table 2.6).[3] The remaining fraction of expenditure growth is due to growth in payments to Medicare and payments to HMOs.

Table 2.6 PERCENTAGE DISTRIBUTION OF MEDICAID EXPENDITURE
GROWTH, BY FACTOR: 1988–92

	Percentage of Total Growth Attributable to Each Factor	
Recipients[a]		36.01
Cash assistance:		8.4
Aged	−0.48	
Blind and Disabled	6.03	
Adults	1.12	
Children	1.69	
Non−cash assistance:		18.4
Aged	9.03	
Blind and Disabled	6.89	
Adults	1.17	
Children	1.27	
New groups (pregnant women and children):		9.30
Adults	3.53	
Children	5.77	
Inflation		25.93
Hospital inpatient	6.16	
Nursing homes	6.43	
Physicians, laboratory, and X-ray	2.13	
Outpatient and clinic	1.46	
Intermediate health care facilities for the mentally retarded	2.42	
Home health	1.33	
Prescription drugs	2.70	
Other	3.32	
Utilization and Reimbursement above Inflation		33.42
Hospital inpatient	21.45	
Nursing homes	0.85	
Physicians, laboratory, and X-ray	1.21	
Outpatient and clinic	3.55	
Intermediate health care facilities for the mentally retarded	−1.55	
Home health	2.88	
Prescription drugs	0.16	
Other	4.86	
Payments to Medicare		2.25
Payments to HMOs		2.39
Total Expenditure Growth		100.00

Note: Arizona and U.S. territories are not included.

a. Recipients represent persons who received any Medicaid service. Those who did not use any service in a given year are not included.

Role of Recipiency Increases

Table 2.6 also shows how—within the three broad categories of recipient growth, inflation, and use and reimbursement above inflation—individual growth factors contributed to total expenditure growth between 1988 and 1992. The top panel displays how increases in the number of recipients affected expenditure growth. We have broken recipients into three main groupings—cash assisted, non–cash-assisted, and pregnant women and children. The cash-assisted are the traditional AFDC and SSI Medicaid recipients, whereas the non–cash-assisted include the medically needy, Qualified Medicare Beneficiaries, and other persons who received Medicaid services but not AFDC or SSI cash grants. The pregnant women and children group comprises individuals who became eligible for Medicaid because of the federal mandates that required states to expand their programs to these populations. These three main recipient groups are then further broken down by eligibility categories—aged, blind and disabled, adults and children.

Increases in the number of Medicaid recipients have been viewed as the single biggest contributor to the recent acceleration in expenditures. Between 1988 and 1992, the Medicaid program experienced exceptionally high enrollment growth: Over that four-year period, the number of recipients swelled from 22.3 million to 29.8 million, an increase of 7.5 million persons (table 2.7). Most of this increase, about 45 percent, was brought about by enrollment of pregnant women and children who became eligible for Medicaid because of the federal mandates. Enrollment of children, cash and non–cash-assisted, accounted for the next largest share of the recipient growth—nearly 25 percent—followed by, in order, the blind and disabled (13.3 percent), adults (11.5 percent), and the aged (5.8 percent). Although overall the number of aged Medicaid recipients increased, the number of cash-assisted elderly actually declined.

Although most of the recipient growth can be attributed to enrollment of newly entitled pregnant women and children, this group accounted for a relatively small share of the spending growth: only 9.3 percent of total Medicaid expenditure increases between 1988 and 1992 was occasioned by the growth of newly covered pregnant women and children (table 2.6). That newly covered pregnant women and children represent a large share of recipient growth but a relatively small share of expenditure growth reflects the fact that this population—particularly children—uses relatively inexpensive

Table 2.7 MEDICAID RECIPIENT GROWTH AND PERCENTAGE OF TOTAL RECIPIENT GROWTH, BY ENROLLMENT GROUP: 1988–92

Recipient[a] Group	Recipients in 1988 (in thousands)	Recipients in 1992 (in thousands)	Average Annual Growth Rates (%)	Share of Total Recipiency Growth (%)
All Groups	22,251	29,795	7.6	100.0
Cash Assistance	16,277	18,538	3.3	30.0
Aged	1,661	1,577	-1.3	-1.1
Blind and disabled	2,745	3,402	5.5	8.7
Adults	3,948	4,385	2.7	5.8
Children	7,923	9,174	3.7	16.6
Non-cash Assistance	5,890	7,761	7.1	24.8
Aged	1,497	2,020	7.8	6.9
Blind and disabled	685	1,030	10.7	4.6
Adults	1,123	1,550	8.4	5.7
Children	2,586	3,160	5.1	7.6
New Groups (Pregnant Women and Children)	84	3,496	153.7	45.2
Adults	44	1,003	118.5	12.7
Children	40	2,493	180.4	32.5

Note: Arizona and U.S. territories are not included.
a. Recipients represent the number of persons who received any Medicaid service. Those who did not use any service in a given year are not included.

health care services as compared to the elderly and the blind and disabled.

The non–cash-assisted accounted for the biggest share of expenditure growth among recipient categories. Nearly 20 percent, or about $11 billion, of overall spending increases resulted from the growth in non–cash-assisted Medicaid recipients—particularly aged and blind and disabled non–cash-assisted recipients. These big spending increases occurred despite the relatively modest growth in the number of non–cash aged and blind and disabled recipients during 1988 to 1992 (table 2.7). As will be discussed further in chapter 6, this irregularity—the low recipient growth coupled with the high expenditure growth—reflects the high costs of long-term care, which is used extensively by the non–cash-assisted elderly and the blind and disabled.

The recipient group that contributed the least to expenditure growth was the cash-assisted, the traditional Medicaid population. Between 1988 and 1992, only about 8.4 percent of spending increases were accounted for by this group (table 2.6). This occurred even though the number of cash-assisted Medicaid recipients increased by more than 2 million over the period.

Role of Medical Care Price Inflation

The second panel of table 2.6, shows how medical care price inflation affected total Medicaid expenditure growth during the 1988–92 period. As mentioned, inflation contributed nearly 26 percent, or about $16 billion, to overall spending increases, suggesting that a large fraction of expenditure growth was economy driven and outside the direct control of the Medicaid program. The bulk of price increases can be attributed to increases for hospital inpatient care and nursing home care. Combined, these two services represented about half of the effect of inflation on overall expenditure growth. However, the contributions of price increases for hospital and nursing home care are somewhat misleading. Because these services account for such a large share of Medicaid spending—about 50 percent—the inflationary effect of hospital and nursing home care reflect more their dollar dominance in the program rather than exceptionally high price increases. In fact, the average annual growth rates in general prices for inpatient hospital care and nursing home care for 1988–92 were among the lowest for major Medicaid services. During that period, based on the price index we developed, prices grew an average of 4.4 percent each year for inpatient hospital care and 5.3 percent for nursing home care. By contrast, growth rates for prescription drugs and physician services were, respectively, 9.4 percent and 6.8 percent.

Role of Use and Reimbursement above Inflation

The third panel of table 2.6 shows the contribution of use and payment above inflation, by service category, to overall expenditure growth. About one-third of total expenditure increases during 1988–92 were accounted for by this category, which includes a compilation of disparate growth factors. For example, this category accounted for expenditure growth due to increased service use among recipients that could have been brought about by utilization of costly new, high-tech medical technologies or by Medicaid recipients consuming more services. It also accounted for spending growth occasioned by recent Boren Amendment-related court decisions that led states to increase provider payment rates. In addition, the category accounted for states' use of special financing programs such as provider tax and disproportionate-share programs.

Nearly two-thirds of the growth in use and payment above inflation can be attributed to reimbursement to inpatient hospitals. In fact, increases in payment to hospitals over inflation was the single largest growth factor, representing an extraordinary 21.5 percent of total expenditure growth, or about $13 billion (table 2.6). Put another way, the contribution of hospital payment growth above inflation to overall spending increases more than doubled that of newly covered pregnant women and children and nearly equaled that of total price inflation.

Role of Special Financing Programs

We suspected that much of the growth in hospital payments was occasioned by states' expanding use of special financing programs, rather than increasing service intensity, Boren Amendment-related litigation, and the like.[4] Beginning in the mid-1980s, many states began to tap a novel gold mine in provider tax and donation programs, and, more recently, intergovernmental transfers programs. Under provider programs, a state would collect such taxes or donations from providers, most often acute care hospitals. Then the state would spend the money and claim federal matching dollars. The most popular mechanism used to spend the money was hospital disproportion-

Table 2.8 PERCENTAGE DISTRIBUTION OF MEDICAID EXPENDITURE GROWTH BY FACTOR, ADJUSTING FOR SPECIAL FINANCING PROGRAMS: 1988–92

	Percentage of Total Growth Attributable to Each Factor		
	Special Revenue[b] Programs Included	Special Revenue[b] Programs Excluded	DSH and Special Revenue[b] Programs Netted Out
Recipients[a]	31.81	36.27	43.98
Cash assistance:	7.4	8.5	10.2
Aged	−0.44	−0.50	−0.61
Blind and disabled	5.43	6.19	7.51
Adults	0.97	1.11	1.34
Children	1.45	1.65	2.00
Non–cash assistance:	17.1	19.6	23.7
Aged	8.75	9.98	12.10
Blind and disabled	6.39	7.29	8.84
Adults	0.97	1.11	1.35
Children	1.03	1.18	1.43
New groups (pregnant women and children):	7.25	8.27	10.02
Adults	2.81	3.20	3.88
Children	4.44	5.06	6.14
Inflation	23.84	27.18	32.96
Hospital inpatient	4.51	5.15	6.24
Nursing homes	6.43	7.33	8.88
Physicians, laboratory, and X-ray	2.13	2.42	2.94
Outpatient and clinic	1.46	1.66	2.02
Intermediate health care facilities for the mentally retarded	2.42	2.76	3.35
Home health	1.33	1.51	1.83
Prescription drugs	2.70	3.07	3.73
Other	2.87	3.28	3.97

	12.05	13.74	16.66
Utilization and Reimbursement above Inflation			
Hospital inpatient	2.99	3.41	4.14
Nursing homes	0.85	0.97	1.18
Physicians, laboratory, and X-ray	1.21	1.38	1.68
Outpatient and clinic	3.55	4.05	4.91
Intermediate health care facilities for the mentally retarded	−1.55	−1.77	−2.15
Home health	2.88	3.29	3.98
Prescription drugs	0.16	0.18	0.22
Other	1.95	2.23	2.70
Payments to Medicare	2.25	2.56	3.10
Payments to HMOs	2.39	2.72	3.30
Special Financing	27.67	17.53	—
Total Expenditure Growth	100.00	100.00	100.00

Note: Arizona and U.S. territories are not included.

a. Recipients represent persons who received any Medicaid service. Those who did not use any service in a given year are not included.

b. Special revenues include provider taxes, provider donations, and intergovernmental transfers.

ate-share (DSH) programs and, more recently, mental health dispro-portionate-share programs.

Intergovernmental transfer programs operate in a comparable fash-ion; that is, local government entities, such as counties or local hospi-tal districts, transfer funds to the state which are subsequently used to claim federal Medicaid matching dollars. For 1992 alone it appears that 38 states collected nearly $8 billion from provider, tax, and intergovernmental transfer programs and that more than $17 billion in DSH payments (both federal and state dollars) were made.

To test whether the bulk of hospital payment growth was caused by increasing use of special financing programs, we reran the decom-position model but added a separate line item that measures how DSH payments affected expenditure growth between 1988 and 1992.[5] These results are shown in table 2.8. According to the model, DSH payments accounted for nearly 27.7 percent of overall Medicaid expenditure growth between 1988 and 1992, making it the second largest overall growth factor. As expected, by separating out DSH payments, the contribution of hospital payments above inflation to overall expenditure growth decreases from 21.5 percent (table 2.6) to 3.0 percent, a percentage in keeping with other major Medicaid services.[6]

Attributing more than a quarter of expenditure growth during 1988–92 to rising DSH payments may be an overestimate. Our DSH estimate counts both federal and state contributions to the payment. Between 1988 and 1992, however, most state contributions to DSH were generated by special revenue programs—provider taxes, dona-tions, and the like—rather than state general funds. Special revenue programs generally functioned so that states contributed no addi-tional state-generated dollars to the programs; instead, states, in essence, temporarily borrowed money from the providers or other entities in order to claim federal matching dollars. Consequently, roughly half of DSH payments (that is, the portion paid by taxes, donations, and transfers) do not represent "true" net increases in payments to providers.

To account for the effect of special financing programs on expendi-ture growth, we ran the decomposition model again but subtracted special financing revenues from DSH payments. To do this, we calcu-lated the ratio of special revenues and total DSH payments. In apply-ing this ratio, we are assuming that all special revenues went to generate federal matching dollars for DSH payments. This may not be entirely accurate, as some of the revenues may have gone for other purposes but, in general, it is a credible assumption.

As shown in the second column of table 2.8, by removing the special financing revenues from the DSH payments, the contribution of DSH payments to overall expenditure growth drops to 17.5 percent. The effects of recipiency growth and price inflation, by contrast, increase. Finally, in the third column we show expenditure growth shares when DSH payments and special revenues are netted out. This column thus shows the role of more traditional growth factors, while assuming that states did not engage in any special financing strategies between 1988 and 1992. Under this assumption, enrollment increases contribute by far the biggest share of expenditure growth, about 44 percent, followed by inflation (33 percent) and use and reimbursement above inflation (17 percent). Among specific enrollment groups, the non–cash-assisted aged and the newly entitled pregnant women and children were the largest contributors. In fact, the former group was the single largest contributor to overall expenditure growth, accounting for 12 percent of total spending increases.

Because of the strong influence of special financing programs on expenditure increases during the 1988–92 period, assigning a share of growth to the various growth factors is not a simple matter. Medicaid hospital inpatient expenditures and inpatient mental health expenditures increased at exceptionally high rates between 1988 and 1992. But whether these expenditures, and what fraction of these expenditures, represent true spending for Medicaid services remains unresolved, and will likely be debated for years to come.

SUMMARY

Since 1981, the spending growth rate for Medicaid has been highly variable. The decade began with a period of relatively slow growth, largely reflecting the impact of OBRA 81. Then in the mid-1980s, the pace of spending growth increased to about 10–13 percent per year. This was occasioned by the introduction of the federal mandates requiring states to expand Medicaid eligibility to new groups such as pregnant women and children. More recently, there has been a rapid escalation in program spending: between 1988 and 1992, total spending for Medicaid grew from $51.4 billion to $112.9 billion, more than 20 percent per year.

A variety of factors contributed to the expenditure surge. An analysis of spending growth between 1988 and 1992, which totaled more than $61 billion, revealed that enrollment increases accounted for

36 percent of the growth. Medical care price inflation accounted for 26 percent of the growth, and use and reimbursement above inflation accounted for another 33 percent. Payments for Medicare and HMOs contributed the remaining fraction.

The recent acceleration in program spending, however, has been heavily influenced by states' increasing use of provider taxes and donations programs, disproportionate-share payments, and intergovernmental transfer programs during 1988–92. Exactly how to account for these programs in terms of their impact on program spending is, at best, difficult. Do they represent true, new spending on Medicaid services? If so, then spending on these programs should be fully counted. Alternatively, if these programs were strictly a way for states to game the federal match, then expenditures for these programs should not be counted. Because of the magnitude of these programs, their effect on expenditure growth patterns is both large and important.

Notes

1. In addition, there are service-specific recipients (those who use a nursing home) and general recipients (those who use any Medicaid service).

2. Unlike the federal matching arrangements with the states, which are annually adjusted on the basis of states' per capita incomes, federal Medicaid matching for the territories are fixed at 50 percent. In addition, overall federal spending caps are put in the territories' Medicaid program.

3. For the decomposition models, we used recipients of any Medicaid services, as opposed to enrollees.

4. As will be discussed in chapter 6, the Boren Amendment, which was first enacted in 1980, sets a federal standard for determining the "reasonableness" of Medicaid reimbursement to hospitals and nursing homes (Anderson and Scanlon 1993). In recent years, the Amendment has been used by providers as a basis to challenge states' payment levels to hospitals and nursing homes.

5. We used two sources of information to compile a record of DSH payments. For 1988, data came from the National Association of Public Hospitals survey of states' DSH programs (National Association of Public Hospitals 1989). The survey estimated that about $500 million DSH payments were made in that year. For 1992, DSH numbers came from the August 1993 HCFA notice on limitations in aggregate payments to disproportionate-share hospitals (*Federal Register* 1993).

6. The contributions of other growth factors also shift somewhat when DSH payments are entered as a separate line item. For example, comparing table 2.5 to table 2.7 shows that the percentage of growth attributed to enrollment declines, going from 36 percent to 32 percent. Likewise, the contributions of medical care price inflation and use and reimbursement above inflation for hospital inpatient car and "other" also decline. The "other" category includes expenditures for inpatient mental health. By 1992,

many states had developed DSH programs for inpatient mental health in addition to inpatient hospital DSH programs. When separating DSH payments, we accounted for both types of DSH programs. (By contrast, the contribution of all services—both for price inflation and use and reimbursement above inflation—do not change when DSH payments were separated out.) The shift in percentages for select growth factors reflects the fact that the relative contribution of hospital inpatient and mental health expenditures to overall growth has declined (with a corresponding rise in growth attributed to DSH payments). Since the decomposition model calculates the shares of expenditure growth for each service for each enrollment group as a product of enrollment growth, medical care price inflation, and use and reimbursement above inflation, then it follows that those growth factors influenced by either inpatient hospital or mental health expenditures should also be affected.

Chapter Three

MEDICAID ELIGIBILITY POLICIES

Eligibility for Medicaid has historically been closely tied to the receipt of cash assistance either through the Aid to Families with Dependent Children (AFDC) program or the Supplemental Security Income (SSI) welfare program. However, starting in the mid-1980s with the passage of the Deficit Reduction Act of 1984, Congress set in motion a series of legislative actions that greatly loosened this tie. In each year between 1984 and 1990, Congress passed at least one major piece of legislation that required, or allowed, states to either expand Medicaid eligibility or services. About half of the eligibility expansions were targeted at pregnant women and children not on AFDC. The other expansions passed during this period extended eligibility to low-income elderly and disabled persons and other specified groups such as newly legalized aliens and the homeless. Collectively, these legislative actions fundamentally changed Medicaid program eligibility, in that an individual no longer has to be receiving welfare to qualify for Medicaid. In 1992, about 60 percent of Medicaid recipients qualified for Medicaid by virtue of being on welfare, down from 80 percent in 1984.

These legislative actions also significantly expanded the number of persons eligible for Medicaid. It has been estimated that over a half-million pregnant women, 4 million to 5 million children, and more than 4 million elderly and disabled individuals have become newly entitled (Rosenbaum 1993).

This chapter examines broad Medicaid eligibility trends and policies since 1981, with a special focus on later years.[1] We begin with a look at the traditional Medicaid populations—the cash assisted and the medically needy. Then we review some of the federal legislation passed during the 1980s that mandated states to expand program eligibility. We highlight legislative initiatives directed at pregnant women and children and the qualified Medicare beneficiary (QMB) mandate (included as part of the 1988 Medicare Catastrophic Cover-

age Act), which required states to help low-income Medicare beneficiaries in paying for Medicare cost sharing. We conclude with an
analysis of how, in the wake of the eligibility expansions, Medicaid's
coverage of the U.S. population has changed over the last decade.

TRADITIONAL MEDICAID POPULATIONS: AFDC AND SSI ENROLLEES AND THE MEDICALLY NEEDY

Medicaid, as mentioned, has long been tightly bound to the cash
welfare system. Although this bond has weakened because of the
recent federal mandates, eligibility for Medicaid remains closely
linked to state and federal welfare policy: to participate in Medicaid,
states, at the least, are required to cover all "categorically needy"
persons, that is, those receiving AFDC and most of those receiving
SSI. Thus, while the AFDC and SSI programs are not formally part
of Medicaid, most changes made to these programs will directly affect
who is eligible for Medicaid.

AFDC and Medicaid

Like Medicaid, AFDC is jointly financed by the states and the federal
government. Typically, families with children become eligible for
AFDC if their incomes and assets fall below predetermined thresholds. Within broad federal rules, states have considerable latitude in
setting these thresholds. One consequence of this flexibility is that
eligibility for AFDC varies greatly across the states: in 1992, the
maximum monthly benefit level for a family of three ranged from a
low of $120 in Mississippi to a high of $924 in Alaska.

Since the early 1980s, it has become increasingly difficult to qualify
for the AFDC program. Between 1980 and 1992, the maximum AFDC
benefit for a family of three declined almost 16 percent in the average
state, after accounting for inflation (table 3.1). The average benefit
level as a percentage of poverty was 46 percent in 1992, down from
54 percent in 1980. In other words, a family with children had to be
considerably poorer in 1992 to qualify for AFDC than it had to be
in 1980.

Over the 1980–92 period, only two states' AFDC benefit levels
increased faster than inflation—Alaska and Georgia. Whereas the
bulk of the states showed large decreases, several showed relatively

Table 3.1 MONTHLY AFDC MAXIMUM BENEFIT LEVEL FOR FAMILY OF
THREE, BY STATE: 1980–92 (CONSTANT 1992 DOLLARS)

State	1980 ($)[a]	1992 ($)	Percentage Change, 1980–92
Alabama	201	149	−25.8
Alaska	778	924	18.7
Arkansas	274	204	−25.6
California	805	663	−17.7
Colorado	494	356	−27.9
Connecticut	809	680	−15.9
Delaware	453	338	−25.4
District of Columbia	487	409	−16.0
Florida	332	303	−8.7
Georgia	279	280	0.3
Hawaii	797	666	−16.4
Idaho	550	315	−42.7
Illinois	490	367	−25.2
Indiana	434	288	−33.7
Iowa	613	426	−30.5
Kansas	587	422	−28.2
Kentucky	320	228	−28.8
Louisiana	259	190	−26.6
Maine	477	453	−5.0
Maryland	460	377	−18.0
Massachusetts	645	539	−16.5
Michigan (Wayne Co.)	724	459	−36.6
Minnesota	710	532	−25.1
Mississippi	163	120	−26.6
Missouri	422	292	−30.8
Montana	441	390	−11.6
Nebraska	528	364	−31.0
Nevada	446	372	−16.6
New Hampshire	589	516	−12.4
New Jersey	613	424	−30.8
New Mexico	397	324	−18.3
New York	671	577	−14.0
North Carolina	327	272	−16.8
North Dakota	569	401	−29.5
Ohio	448	334	−25.4
Oklahoma	480	341	−29.0
Oregon	576	460	−20.1
Pennsylvania	565	421	−25.5
Rhode Island	579	554	−4.3
South Carolina	220	210	−4.4
South Dakota	547	404	−26.1
Tennessee	208	185	−10.9
Texas	198	184	−6.8

(continued)

Table 3.1 MONTHLY AFDC MAXIMUM BENEFIT LEVEL FOR FAMILY OF
THREE, BY STATE: 1980–92 (CONSTANT 1992 DOLLARS) (*continued*)

State	1980 ($)[a]	1992 ($)	Percentage Change, 1980–92
Utah	613	402	− 34.4
Vermont	838	673	− 19.7
Virginia	528	354	− 32.9
Washington	780	531	− 31.9
West Virginia	351	249	− 29.0
Wisconsin	756	517	− 31.6
Wyoming	536	360	− 32.9
Weighted mean[b]	506	425	− 15.9
Mean benefit as percentage of poverty	54.3%	45.6%	− 16.0
Coefficient of variation	42.3%	39.0%	− 7.8

Source: U.S. Congress, House Committee on Ways and Means (henceforth, Committee on Ways and Means) (1993).
a. The Consumer Price Index-Urban (CPI-U) was used to inflate 1980 benefit levels to 1992 levels.
b. Weighted by average monthly number of AFDC recipients by state.

modest declines in benefit levels, such as Florida, Maine, Rhode Island, South Carolina, and Texas. AFDC payment levels among the states remained as varied in 1992 as they had been in 1980, as indicated by the coefficient of variation in the two years (see table 3.1).[2]

That AFDC benefit levels fall so far below the poverty line can be attributed partly to the fact that there is no set minimum AFDC standard required by the federal government; determining program standards is mostly left to the states' discretion. Low benefit levels can also be attributed to the recent budget-cutting efforts by states, which have hit the AFDC program particularly hard. In 1992, for example, 44 states either froze or cut AFDC benefits (Lav et al. 1993). These reductions often followed similar cuts in 40 states in 1991.

Despite increasingly restrictive AFDC eligibility standards, the number of people enrolled in the program has recently begun to accelerate. After many years of little to no growth, the number of families enrolled in AFDC rose from 4 million to nearly 4.8 million between 1990 and 1992 (table 3.2). This corresponds to an increase of more than 2 million individuals receiving AFDC payments. Much of this growth can be attributed to the rising number of families receiving *basic* AFDC assistance. (We use the term basic to describe those AFDC families who have historically been covered under Medicaid; that is, single-parent families with children.) After an extended

Table 3.2 AVERAGE MONTHLY AFDC ENROLLMENTS: 1981–92
(NUMBER OF FAMILIES IN THOUSANDS)

Fiscal Year(s)	Total	AFDC-UP	AFDC Basic
1981	3,871	209	3,662
1984	3,725	287	3,438
1987	3,784	236	3,548
1990	3,967	203	3,764
1992	4,769	322	4,447
Average Annual Growth Rates:			
1981–84	− 1.3%	11.2%	− 2.1%
1984–87	0.5	− 6.3	1.1
1987–90	1.6	− 4.9	2.0
1990–92	9.6	25.9	8.7
1981–92	1.9	4.0	1.8

Source: Committee on Ways and Means (1993).

period of virtually no increases, there has been a recent surge in basic AFDC enrollment: the number of basic AFDC families grew from 3.8 million families in 1990 to 4.4 million in 1992, about a 9 percent annual increase.

Most likely, the recent recession caused much of this growth. The expanding number of female-headed households in the United States may be another contributing factor (Congressional Budget Office 1992). The new Medicaid outreach efforts, such as streamlining Medicaid eligibility and "outstationing" eligibility workers (that is, placing them where potential AFDC recipients receive medical care, as opposed to the welfare office) may have also contributed to the AFDC enrollment growth. Although such efforts did not increase the number of persons eligible for AFDC, individuals applying for Medicaid may have learned they were also entitled to AFDC benefits. A recent study, for instance, has shown that the new Medicaid outreach programs have had a marked impact on Food Stamp Program participation rates (McConnell 1991).

Whereas increases in basic enrollees account for the bulk of the recent surge in AFDC enrollment, the rate of growth in a category of enrollees known as "AFDC-UP" families has been significantly higher. Unlike basic AFDC families, AFDC-UP families are two-parent families in which one principal breadwinner is unemployed. Between 1990 and 1992, the average monthly AFDC-UP enrollment grew some 26 percent each year (table 3.2), a growth rate that can be attributed to passage of the Family Support Act (FSA) of 1988, which required states to provide AFDC coverage to families who are in need because the principal wage earner is unemployed. Families covered by the FSA are commonly referred to as AFDC-UP. Before 1988, coverage of AFDC-UP families was an optional benefit provided by 31 states. Since AFDC-UP expressly covers unemployed persons, the impact of the FSA has been particularly strong because its enactment directly preceded the recession of the early 1990s.

SSI and Medicaid

Supplemental Security Income, or SSI, provides cash assistance to poor aged and disabled persons. As mentioned, to participate in the Medicaid program, states are required, with a few exceptions, to cover SSI recipients. Most states extend Medicaid coverage to all SSI recipients. However, 12 states, commonly referred to as 209(b) states after a section in the Social Security Amendments of 1972, use a separate set of Medicaid eligibility policies for SSI recipients that may be more restrictive than SSI eligibility policies. Consequently, in some 209(b) states persons can receive SSI cash grants but not be eligible for Medicaid.

Unlike AFDC or Medicaid, the basic SSI program is funded entirely by the federal government. Income and asset eligibility standards for the SSI program are set nationally and adjusted each year for inflation. In addition, states are allowed to supplement the basic federal SSI grant with state supplemental payments (SSPs), which are set and funded in full by state funds. In 1992, 27 states elected to provide SSPs to their SSI recipients. Among states, the level of payment varied greatly, from $2 in Oregon to $374 in Alaska; the median payment was $32. Under Medicaid law, states that elect to provide SSPs are given the option to offer the same Medicaid coverage to SSP recipients as they extend to SSI recipients. In general, most states exercise this option.

The 1992 basic federal SSI benefit for an elderly individual who lived alone was $422, or 75 percent of the federal poverty line. When state supplemental payments are counted, the mean weighted benefit level in that year was $482 (table 3.3). Since the federal SSI payment is determined for the nation and annually adjusted for cost of living, the effects of inflation over time on SSI benefits have not been as dramatic as they have been for AFDC. The average state SSI/SSP benefit for an elderly person living alone basically kept pace with inflation over the 1980–92 time period.

Because the federal SSI grant is so large relative to state SSPs,

Table 3.3 MONTHLY SSI/SSP BENEFIT LEVEL FOR SINGLE ELDERLY PERSON
LIVING ALONE, BY STATE: 1980–92 (CONSTANT 1992 DOLLARS)

State	1980 ($)[a]	1992 ($)	Percentage Change, 1980–92
Alabama	405	422	4.1
Alaska	805	784	−2.7
Arkansas	405	422	4.1
California	684	645	−5.8
Colorado	499	478	−4.2
Connecticut	405	747	84.3
Delaware	405	422	4.1
District of Columbia	431	437	1.4
Florida	405	422	4.1
Georgia	405	422	4.1
Hawaii	431	427	−0.9
Idaho	531	492	−7.4
Illinois	405	422	4.1
Indiana	405	422	4.1
Iowa	405	422	4.1
Kansas	405	422	4.1
Kentucky	405	422	4.1
Louisiana	405	422	4.1
Maine	422	432	2.3
Maryland	405	422	4.1
Massachusetts	639	551	−13.7
Michigan	446	436	−2.3
Minnesota	463	503	8.6
Mississippi	405	422	4.1
Missouri	405	422	4.1
Montana	405	422	4.1
Nebraska	533	452	−15.2
Nevada	485	458	−5.6
New Hampshire	484	449	−7.1
New Jersey	444	453	1.9
New Mexico	405	422	4.1
New York	513	508	−0.9
North Carolina	405	422	4.1
North Dakota	405	422	4.1
Ohio	405	422	4.1
Oklahoma	540	486	−10.0
Oregon	426	424	−0.4
Pennsylvania	460	454	−1.2
Rhode Island	477	489	2.6
South Carolina	405	422	4.1
South Dakota	431	437	1.4
Tennessee	405	422	4.1
Texas	405	422	4.1

(continued)

Table 3.3 MONTHLY SSI/SSP BENEFIT LEVEL FOR SINGLE ELDERLY PERSON
LIVING ALONE, BY STATE: 1980–92 (CONSTANT 1992 DOLLARS)
(*continued*)

State	1980 ($)[a]	1992 ($)	Percentage Change, 1980–92
Utah	422	427	1.1
Vermont	475	487	2.5
Virginia	405	422	4.1
Washington	478	450	−5.9
West Virginia	405	422	4.1
Wisconsin	576	514	−10.7
Wyoming	439	442	0.6
Weighted mean[b]	484	482	−0.4
Mean benefit as percentage of poverty	86.3%	85.6%	−0.8
Coefficient of variation	22.2%	17.9%	−19.3

Source: Committee on Ways and Means (1993).
a. The CPI-U was used to inflate 1980 benefit levels to 1992 levels.
b. Weighted by number of SSI recipients.

evaluating the two together masks some changes that have been made
to SSP levels by states. Between 1980 and 1992, the median state
supplemental payment declined by 55 percent, after adjusting for
inflation. Like most other state budget items, SSP has also been cut
in recent years. Although not usually a large state budget item, SSPs
are funded entirely by state dollars. Consequently, each dollar cut
in SSPs translates into a dollar saved for the state. In 1991, five states
cut their SSPs, followed by four more states in 1992. This trend
contrasts with earlier periods, when it was rare for states to actually
cut SSPs, although freezing of payments did occur (Lav et al.1993).

Between 1981 and 1992, the number of persons receiving SSI rose
gradually, increasing about 3 percent each year (table 3.4). This
increase is entirely accounted for by the growth in the number of
blind and disabled persons receiving SSI payments, whereas the
number of aged persons on SSI has declined since the early 1980s.
Although the number of blind and disabled SSI recipients expanded
steadily during this period, growth for this group has been particularly rapid since 1990, increasing 10.3 percent per year. Several factors have contributed to the recent enrollment surge. Although not
reflected in table 3.4, much of the growth was caused by increases
in the number of disabled SSI children, a growth that was occasioned
by the 1990 Supreme Court decision *Sullivan v. Zebley*, which

Table 3.4 NUMBER OF PERSONS RECEIVING FEDERALLY ADMINISTERED SSI
PAYMENTS: 1981–92 (IN THOUSANDS)

Fiscal Year(s)	Total	Aged	Blind or Disabled
1981	4,019	1,678	2,341
1984	4,029	1,530	2,499
1987	4,385	1,455	2,930
1990	4,817	1,454	3,363
1992	5,566	1,471	4,095
Average Annual Growth Rates:			
1981–84	0.1%	− 3.0%	2.2%
1984–87	2.9	− 1.7	5.4
1987–90	3.2	0.0	4.7
1990–92	7.5	0.6	10.3
1981–92	3.0	− 1.2	5.2

Source: Committee on Ways and Means (1993).

required the U.S. Social Security Administration to conduct retroactive eligibility determinations back to 1980 for disabled children[3] (Sullivan v. Zebley, 1990). This decision alone added about 125,000 new SSI recipients (Congressional Research Service 1992).

Another factor that has contributed to the swelling number of disabled SSI recipients is the increase in the number of people applying for benefits and the corresponding growth in the number of applications approved by the Social Security Administration (Congressional Budget Office 1992). Exactly why this has happened is not clear, but it stems partly from the movement among advocacy groups for the disabled to educate their constituents about available benefits.

Acquired immunodeficiency syndrome (AIDS) may also be a contributing factor. As life spans of persons with AIDS are extended owing to improvements in medical treatments for the disease, the number of disabled people with AIDS who qualify for SSI is likely increasing. In addition, beginning in 1991, the Social Security Administration implemented a new regulation allowing for presumptive disability for persons with human immunodeficiency virus (HIV), thus enabling them to qualify for SSI benefits. Previously, only those diagnosed with AIDS qualified.

As stated, although the number of disabled SSI recipients has been growing, aged enrollment has been steadily declining: from 1981 to 1992, the number of elderly SSI beneficiaries decreased by more than twelve percent. This trend reflects the declining rate of poverty among the aged, a trend that began in the 1960s.

The Medically Needy and Medicaid

Beyond covering AFDC and SSI recipients, states also have the option to extend Medicaid coverage to the "medically needy." Eligibility under this option is also tied to the welfare system: the medically needy are individuals who meet all the categorical criteria for either the AFDC or the SSI programs (for example, they are aged, blind, or pregnant) and have income and asset levels that fall below medically needy program standards, after deducting their medical expenses. If a state elects to offer the medically needy option, it can extend coverage to all categorically eligible groups, but it must cover pregnant women and children. Most states provide coverage to other groups, particularly the aged and the blind and disabled, who generally meet the medically needy financial criteria by spending-down their income and assets because of high institutional care costs.

In 1992, 36 states and the District of Columbia had medically needy programs. All but one state, Texas, covered the aged and the blind and disabled. In fact, the medically needy option over time has evolved into a program that serves principally these populations, particularly the institutionalized elderly. (Although most states with medically needy programs covered institutional care for the aged, not all did. In 1992, 29 out of the 36 states with medically needy programs offered such care.) Because of the new federal mandates requiring states to extend Medicaid protection to low-income pregnant women and children, the medically needy option will, in the future, likely become almost exclusively dedicated to the elderly and the blind and disabled.

To qualify for medically needy coverage, a person must first deplete his or her income and resources to specified levels. Income eligibility thresholds are determined by the states and can be set up to one-third higher than the state's maximum AFDC benefit level. Because of this close link to the AFDC program, there is considerable variability in medically needy standards across the states. Another consequence of this close tie to the AFDC program is that medially needy standards are often below those for the SSI program. In 1992, standards ranged from a low of $301 in Texas to a high of $1,100 in California (table 3.5).

Between 1980 and 1992, the medically needy program both expanded and contracted. Several states, for example, elected to begin providing medically needy protection: Florida, Georgia, Iowa, New Jersey, Oregon, South Carolina, and Texas all began to extend medically needy coverage to their residents. Some states also expanded

Table 3.5 MONTHLY MEDICALLY NEEDY NEED STANDARD FOR FAMILY OF
FOUR, BY STATE: 1980–92 (CONSTANT 1992 DOLLARS)

State	1980 ($)[a]	1992 ($)[b]	Percentage Change, 1980–92
Alabama	—	—	—
Alaska	—	—	—
Arkansas	440	333	− 24.3
California	1,107	1,100	− 0.6
Colorado	—	—	—
Connecticut[a]	851	908	6.7
Delaware	—	—	—
District of Columbia	690	665	− 3.6
Florida	—	364	N.A.
Georgia	—	442	N.A.
Hawaii	936	802	− 14.4
Idaho	—	—	—
Illinois	567	558	− 1.6
Indiana	—	—	—
Iowa	—	666	N.A.
Kansas	698	488	− 30.1
Kentucky	539	383	− 29.0
Louisiana[c]	497	317	− 36.2
Maine	809	575	− 28.9
Maryland	582	484	− 16.9
Massachusetts	749	891	18.9
Michigan[c]	850	593	− 30.3
Minnesota	753	828	10.0
Mississippi	—	—	—
Missouri	—	—	—
Montana	993	469	− 52.8
Nebraska	1,022	584	− 42.8
Nevada	—	—	—
New Hampshire	810	623	− 23.1
New Jersey	—	658	N.A.
New Mexico	—	—	—
New York	922	850	− 7.8
North Carolina	568	400	− 29.5
North Dakota	1,132	530	− 53.2
Ohio	—	—	—
Oklahoma	1,064	567	− 46.7
Oregon	—	753	N.A.
Pennsylvania	837	567	− 32.3
Rhode Island	1,234	850	− 31.1
South Carolina	—	341	N.A.
South Dakota	—	—	—
Tennessee	468	308	− 34.2
Texas	—	301	N.A.

(continued)

Table 3.5 MONTHLY MEDICALLY NEEDY NEED STANDARD FOR FAMILY OF
FOUR, BY STATE: 1980–92 (CONSTANT 1992 DOLLARS) (continued)

State	1980 ($)[a]	1992 ($)[b]	Percentage Change, 1980–92
Utah	1,187	626	−47.3
Vermont[c]	1,051	1,008	−4.1
Virginia[c]	809	400	−50.5
Washington	1,178	725	−38.5
West Virginia	610	312	−48.8
Wisconsin	1,234	823	−33.3
Wyoming	—	—	—
Weighted mean[d]	849	654	−22.9
Mean state as percentage of poverty	71.1%	54.8%	−23.0
Coefficient of variation	28.5%	44.3%	55.6

Notes: N.A., Not applicable; dash (—) denotes no medically needy program.
a. From Health Care Financing Administration, 1981, *Program Statistics: Medicare and Medicaid Data Book* (Washington, D.C.: U.S. Government Printing Office).
b. Congressional Research Service, 1993, *Medicaid Source Book: Background Data and Analysis. A 1993 Update* (Washington, D.C.: U.S. Government Printing Office). The CPI-U was used to inflate 1980 standard levels to 1992 levels.
c. In 1980 highest regional level is used.
d. Weighted by number of SSI recipients.

medically needy coverage to groups other than pregnant women and children. At the same time, after accounting for inflation, the medically needy standard declined an average of 23 percent over the period, more than the average decline in AFDC benefit level (table 3.5). In 1992 the mean monthly medically needy standard was 55 percent of poverty, down from 71 percent in 1980. Although the bulk of the states did not keep pace with the cost of living, standards in three states (Connecticut, Massachusetts, and Minnesota) actually grew at rates faster than inflation. Finally, medically needy standards became more diverse among the states between 1980 and 1992, as indicated by the increase in the coefficient of variation in the two years (see table 3.5).

To summarize, Medicaid was established to provide health care to the poor, principally those receiving cash assistance. Although SSI financial eligibility criteria have kept pace with inflation over the 1980–92 time period, criteria for the other two traditional Medicaid populations—AFDC and medically needy—have become increasingly restrictive: After adjusting for the cost of living, qualifying income levels for AFDC recipients have generally declined by nearly

16 percent, and by nearly 23 percent for the medically needy. Thus, for these populations, access to Medicaid has substantially eroded since 1980.

MEDICAID ELIGIBILITY EXPANSIONS

In an effort to stem this erosion, beginning in the mid-1980s Congress enacted a series of mandates and options that greatly increased states' ability to extend Medicaid's coverage to specific populations. As noted, although most of these legislative expansions were targeted at pregnant women and children, they also affected other populations, including the aged, the blind and disabled, newly legalized aliens, and the homeless (table 3.6). Within a short time, the pool of persons eligible for Medicaid greatly enlarged, owing to these congressional actions. This section reviews two important eligibility expansions: those directed at pregnant women and children and the qualified Medicare beneficiary (QMB) mandates, which required states to help low-income Medicare beneficiaries with Medicare cost sharing.

Pregnant Women and Children Eligibility Mandates and Options

Over the last several years, Congress has greatly liberalized Medicaid eligibility policies for pregnant women and children: between 1984 and 1990, Medicaid law was amended 10 times to expand program coverage to these groups. The major motivating factors for these legislative actions came from states' growing concern about eroding health care coverage among poor children and high infant mortality rates. In particular, the southern states—with a high incidence of low-birthweight babies and high infant mortality rates as well as low Medicaid eligibility thresholds—spearheaded the campaign to expand Medicaid coverage of pregnant women and children.

Within a short period, these congressional mandates and options greatly altered Medicaid eligibility rules and procedures for pregnant women and children. Initially, under the Deficit Reduction Act of 1984, states were required to expand Medicaid coverage to pregnant women and children who met the AFDC income and resource eligibility limits but whose family structure made them ineligible for AFDC. For example, states were mandated to provide benefits to pregnant women who met AFDC standards but had no other children.

Table 3.6 MAJOR FEDERAL EXPANSIONS OF MEDICAID ELIGIBILITY: 1984–90

Legislation	Population Affected	Expansion
DEFRA 1984 (Deficit Reduction Act of 1984, P.L. 98-369)	Infants[a] and children	Requires coverage of all children born after 9/30/83 meeting state AFDC income and resource standards, regardless of family structure.
	Pregnant women	Requires coverage from date of medical verification of pregnancy, providing: (1) they would qualify for AFDC once child was born or (2) they would qualify for AFDC-UP[b] once child was born, regardless of whether state has AFDC-UP program.
	Infants	Requires automatic coverage for one year after birth if mother already is receiving Medicaid and remains eligible, and infant resides with her.
COBRA 1985 (Consolidated Omnibus Budget Reconciliation Act of 1985, P.L. 99-272)	Pregnant women	Requires coverage if family income and resources below state AFDC levels, regardless of family structure.
	Postpartum women	Requires 60-day extension of coverage postpartum if eligibility was pregnancy-related. Allows extension of DEFRA coverage up to age five immediately, instead of requiring phase-in by birth date.
	Adoptive and foster children	Requires coverage even if adoption/foster agreement was entered into in another state.

OBRA 1986 (Omnibus Budget Reconciliation Act of 1986, P.L. 99-509)	Aged and disabled	Creates new optional categorically needy group for those with income below 100 percent of poverty under certain resource constraints. Option can be exercised for this group only if exercised also for pregnant women and infants.
	Aged and disabled	Allows Medicare buy-in[c] up to 100 percent of poverty for qualified Medicare beneficiaries under certain resource constraints.
	Pregnant women and infants	Creates new optional categorically needy group for those with income below 100 percent of poverty. Women receive pregnancy-related services only. Allows assets test to be dropped for this newly defined category of applicants. Allows presumptive eligibility for up to 45 days to be determined by qualified provider. Allows guarantee of continuous eligibility through postpartum period.
	Children	Allows coverage up to age five, if income below 100 percent of poverty (phased in).
	Severely impaired	Established new mandatory categorically needy coverage group for qualified individuals under age 65.
	Aliens	Requires provision of emergency services if otherwise eligible (financially and categorically).

(continued)

Table 3.6 MAJOR FEDERAL EXPANSIONS OF MEDICAID ELIGIBILITY: 1984–90   (continued)

Legislation	Population Affected	Expansion
IRCA 1986 (Immigration Reform and Control Act of 1986, P.L. 99-603)	Newly legalized aliens	Requires provision of emergency and pregnancy-related services if otherwise eligible. Also requires full coverage for eligibles under age 18.
Anti-Drug Abuse Act 1986 (P.L. 99-570)	Homeless	Requires states to provide proof of eligibility for individuals otherwise eligible but having no permanent address.
OBRA 1987 (Omnibus Budget Reconciliation Act of 1987, P.L. 100-203)	Pregnant women and infants	Allows coverage if income level below 185 percent of poverty.
	Children	Allows immediate extension of OBRA 1986 coverage up to 100 percent of poverty up to age five. Allows coverage for children aged five to seven, up to state AFDC level (phased in by age). Allows coverage for children below age nine, up to 100 percent of poverty (phased in by age).
MCCA (Medicare Catastrophic Coverage Act of 1988, P.L. 100-360)	Pregnant women and infants	Requires coverage up to 100 percent of poverty (phased in by percentage of poverty).
	Elderly and disabled	Requires Medicare buy-in up to 100 percent of poverty for QMBs (phased in by percentage of poverty).
Family Support Act of 1988 (P.L. 100-485)	AFDC families with unemployed parent (AFDC-UP)	Requires coverage if otherwise qualified.

OBRA 1989 (Omnibus Budget Reconciliation Act of 1989, P.L. 101-239)	Pregnant women and infants	Requires coverage if income is below 133 percent of poverty.
	Children	Requires coverage up to age six, up to 133 percent of poverty.
OBRA 1990 (Omnibus Budget Reconciliation Act of 1990, P.L. 101-508)	Children	Requires coverage up to age 18, if income is below 100 percent of poverty (phased in by age).
	Pregnant women	Requires continuous eligibility through postpartum period.
	Pregnant women and children	Requires states to receive and process applications at convenient outreach sites.
	Infants	Requires continuous eligibility if (1) born to Medicaid-eligible mother who would remain eligible if pregnant and (2) remaining in mother's household.
	Elderly and disabled	Extends MCCA QMB provision to 120 percent of poverty (phased in by percentage of poverty).

Source: U.S. General Accounting Office (1991).

a. Infants are children up to age one.

b. AFDC-UP allows coverage in two-parent families if principal wage earner is unemployed.

c. Medicaid covers Medicare cost-sharing charges: premiums, deductibles, and coinsurance.

Previously, a pregnant woman could receive Medicaid only if she had other children.

Then, Congress, in the Omnibus Budget Reconciliation Act of 1986 (OBRA 86), gave states the option to extend Medicaid benefits to pregnant women and infants with incomes above the AFDC standard but below 100 percent of the federal poverty level without regard to family structure. This same option was also extended to children on an incremental basis. In addition, OBRA 86 allowed states to waive the asset test for Medicaid eligibility; that is, states could base eligibility on income alone for the newly entitled groups. It was OBRA 86 that began to loosen the strong, historical link between Medicaid and AFDC. Moreover, with passage of this legislation, states could expand Medicaid coverage to low-income women and children without increasing AFDC payments.

Later, as part of OBRA 87, states were given the option to cover pregnant women and infants below 185 percent of poverty. OBRA 87 also allowed states to accelerate the coverage of children included as part of OBRA 86 (that is, children ages five and under). In addition, OBRA 87 gave states the option to cover older poor children up to age nine.

In the following year, the Medicare Catastrophic Coverage Act (MCCA) of 1988 mandated that states cover pregnant women and infants with income up to 100 percent of poverty on an incremental basis. (Previously, states had been allowed, but not required, to provide this coverage.) This coverage was later expanded, by OBRA 89, so that all pregnant women and children up to age six in families with incomes below 133 percent of poverty were entitled to Medicaid benefits. In the next year, OBRA 90 mandated that states phase in coverage of children up to age 18 living in poverty. In addition, OBRA 90 made some relatively minor changes in eligibility for pregnant women.

In general, states enthusiastically embraced these eligibility mandates and options principally because they were concerned about infant mortality and poor child health. In addition, the mandates provided federal matching dollars for the services provided to newly entitled groups, services that previously had been funded primarily with state dollars. Besides complying with the mandates (often before they became mandatory), many states took full advantage of the optional provisions. For example, OBRA 89, as noted, required states to cover pregnant women and infants up to 133 percent of the poverty line, but allowed them to cover those with incomes up to 185 percent of poverty. By 1992, 31 states exceeded the minimum coverage level and 25 states elected to provide the highest optional coverage. Some states have also gone beyond the minimum eligibility levels for children, although not to the same extent as they have for pregnant women and infants.

Beyond the eligibility expansions themselves, states also rapidly adopted a number of congressional options that were designed to help implement the expansions. These included granting "presumptive eligibility" for Medicaid coverage to pregnant women while their applications were being processed and the earlier-mentioned "outstationing" of Medicaid eligibility workers. These efforts, which sought to both encourage enrollment and ease the application process, apparently have been successful, and particularly for women: A 1991 General Accounting Office study reported that up to three-quarters of newly entitled pregnant women had enrolled in Medicaid (U.S. General Accounting Office 1991).

Beyond successfully enrolling pregnant women, the Medicaid program appears to be financing an increasing share of births in the United States. In a 1991 telephone survey, the Children's Defense Fund found that up to 45 percent of all births are now being paid for by Medicaid. Other studies have suggested that such coverage may be higher still in some states (Dubay et al. 1993; Holahan et al. 1992). By contrast, in 1985, before the expansions took hold, Medicaid paid for an estimated 17 percent of all births (Gold, Kenney, and Singh 1987).

Whereas enrollment of pregnant women and infants has been swift, enrollment of children, those aged one and older, has been much slower. A variety of reasons may be contributing to this slow growth. Typically, children enroll in Medicaid when they need health care. Most children, however, do not require care unless they are ill. Consequently, in general, children's contact with the health care system is likely to be less than it is for pregnant women (Rosenbaum 1993). In addition, children's health care costs, on average, are comparatively less than those for pregnant women. This may lower the incentive for families to seek Medicaid coverage for their children for routine health care. Finally, there is some evidence that the same level of community outreach (for example, outstationing of eligibility workers) that is being done to recruit pregnant women is not being extended to children (Rosenbaum 1993).

Although it seems clear that states readily adopted and implemented the expansionary mandates (at least for pregnant women), the health impact of the mandates is not yet known. Early studies have reported mixed findings. An evaluation of expanded Medicaid coverage for pregnant women in Tennessee, for example, reported that after broadening coverage of pregnant women from 45 percent of poverty to 100 percent of poverty, enrollment increased and the share of women who received no prenatal care or did not begin such care until the third trimester significantly declined (Piper et al. 1992). However, the study found no marked improvement in the rates of very low- or moderately low-birthweight children, or of infant mortality. Similar findings were reported in a recent evaluation of Washington State's pregnant women eligibility expansions (Connell 1992).

Qualified Medicare Beneficiary Mandates

The qualified Medicare beneficiary (QMB) mandate was included as part of the 1988 Medicare Catastrophic Cost Act (MCCA). MCCA was, in part, enacted in response to concerns that out-of-pocket costs associated with Medicare cost sharing were becoming increasingly burdensome for poor and low-income Medicare beneficiaries. For most covered services, Medicare charges both a deductible and coinsurance. In addition, to participate in Medicare Part B, which provides physician coverage, Medicare charges a monthly premium. Throughout the 1980s, legislative changes to Medicare substantially increased enrollees' average cost sharing for Medicare services (Moon 1993). While most Medicare beneficiaries purchase private insurance to fill the "gaps" in Medicare coverage, for poor and low-income beneficiaries such insurance is often unaffordable.

The QMB mandate required that, on a phased-in basis, states pay Medicare premiums and cost-sharing charges for Medicare beneficiaries with incomes below the poverty level and assets less than twice the SSI resource level. Specifically, Medicaid pays the Medicare Part B monthly premium, Medicare Part A monthly premium, and coinsurance, and deductibles under both Parts A and B. This protection was extended to both aged and disabled Medicare beneficiaries. Beneficiaries eligible for this protection are commonly referred to as QMBs. Medicaid is limited to paying for these specific charges, unless the individual is entitled to Medicaid otherwise.

Since Medicaid's inception, states have been allowed to "buy-in" Medicare Part B coverage for eligible Medicaid beneficiaries. Under buy-in agreements, Medicaid was responsible for the Part B premium, coinsurance, and deductibles whereas Medicare was responsible for provider reimbursement under its usual coverage and payment rules. Virtually all states had a buy-in agreement for at least some of its eligible Medicaid beneficiaries. In addition to buy-in protection, states have also had the option to provide full Medicaid coverage to elderly and disabled Medicare beneficiaries with incomes below poverty since 1986; only six states though had exercised this option prior to the passage of the MCCA.[4]

The Omnibus Budget Reconciliation Act of 1990 extended the QMB mandate by requiring states on an incremental basis to pay Medicare Part B premiums for near-poor beneficiaries; that is, persons whose incomes exceeded the poverty level. By 1995, Medicaid will cover Part B premiums for those with incomes below 120 percent of poverty. For the near-poor, Medicaid will cover Part B premiums only; coinsurance and deductibles are not included. Persons covered under this mandate are commonly referred to as specified low-income Medicare beneficiaries or SLIMBs.

Unlike the pregnant women and children mandates, states have been reluctant to adopt the QMB mandates. The precise number of QMBs is not known (largely because of state reporting errors), but some evidence exists that enrollment has been slow. A 1993 study, for example, reported that the QMB program had enrolled only about half of the estimated 4 million QMB-eligible elderly persons (Families USA 1993). (The study did not report the coverage of poor disabled Medicare beneficiaries who were also entitled to the QMB benefit.) Medicare claims data from 1992 suggested that coverage may be lower still (Congressional Research Service 1993).

The principal reason for states' lack of enthusiasm is that they believe the federal government itself should be providing the protections covered by the mandates (Holahan et al. 1992). That is, from the states' perspective, the QMB mandates requiring the Medicaid program to cover gaps in the Medicare program is the federal government's responsibility, not the states'. In 1991, the National Governors' Association called for the repeal of the QMB provisions.

Medicaid and Coverage of the Poor

How well does Medicaid cover the poor? This question takes on particular importance because of the recent series of federal mandates requiring states to expand Medicaid eligibility. Using data from the March Current Population Survey (CPS) of the U.S. Bureau of the Census, we evaluated broad insurance coverage trends in this section. With a special focus on Medicaid, we analyzed shifts in health insurance coverage that have occurred between 1984 and 1991.[5] (In the CPS, health care coverage refers to enrollment in an insurance plan; it does not mean service recipiency.)

Over the years, changes have been made to the CPS that affect survey estimates. Specifically, changes made in the March 1988 survey were important to our analysis. These revisions primarily affected the comprehensiveness of health insurance information for children, young adults, and retirees. In brief, before the 1988 survey, children and young adults whose insurance coverage came from a policyholder who lived outside the surveyed household were incorrectly counted as being uninsured. Prior to 1988, the CPS also failed to account for children's health coverage that was independent of adult coverage. Moreover, before 1988 retirees were not asked about their employment-related health benefits. These problems were fixed in the 1988 CPS, with the net effect being that there is a drop in the number of uninsured persons between 1987 and 1988 as recorded by the CPS.[6]

Although the 1988 CPS improved estimates of health care coverage, data before 1988 are not directly comparable to those obtained after 1988. Since we were interested in insurance patterns dating back to the early 1980s, we tried to correct for some of the survey inconsistencies by presenting post-1988 data in two versions: including and excluding "cover-sheet children." Cover-sheet children refers to those children whose health insurance coverage was determined by the new questions added to the "cover sheet" of the 1988 survey (for example, children identified as having insurance because of non-household policyholder or because of employment). Excluding cover-sheet children from the 1988–92 survey data accounts for some of the differences between the pre- and post-1988 surveys, but not all of them. Thus, when data both before and after 1988 are present, some inconsistencies still remain.

A final caveat: When CPS estimates are compared to program administrative data for Medicaid and other welfare programs (such as AFDC, SSI, and Food Stamps), it is apparent that survey respondents underreport their use of such programs. A recently completed study, for example, found that the number of nonelderly, noninstitutionalized persons reporting Medicaid coverage on the March 1991 CPS was 21 percent lower than the unduplicated counts reported in the Health Care Financing Administration's report, HCFA-2082 (Winterbottom 1993). In addition, the CPS also underestimates Medicaid coverage rates because persons living in institutions are not sampled; by contrast, HCFA data account for such individuals. Because of underreporting and sample design, the CPS Medicaid coverage data reported here are lower than those reported elsewhere in the book, which rely on HCFA-2082 data.

To determine an individual's health care coverage, we arranged the various types of coverage categories in a hierarchy, with Medicaid at the top followed by employer-based insurance, other public insurance, own private insurance, and uninsured. Thus, persons who indicated that they had more than one type of health insurance during the year were placed in the first appropriate category.[7] If an individual, for example, indicated receiving both Medicaid and Medicare, he or she was placed in the Medicaid insurance group.

Expanding Medicaid Coverage, Rising Uninsured, Declining Employer-Based Coverage

Tables 3.7 and 3.8 show health insurance coverage rates for the whole population, the poor, and the near-poor as estimated by the CPS. The first table documents coverage rates when cover-sheet children are not included; the second shows rates when these children are included. The proportion of the population covered by Medicaid has been growing: excluding cover-sheet children, in 1991 nearly 10 percent of the population was covered by Medicaid, up from 8.3 percent in 1984 (table 3.7). Including cover-sheet children, the fraction of the population insured by Medicaid increased from 8.5 percent in 1988 to 10.7 percent in 1991 (table 3.8).

Among the poor, Medicaid coverage has substantially increased. Between 1984 and 1991, the share of the poor population—those with incomes below the federal poverty line—protected by Medicaid increased by more than 4 percentage points, excluding cover-sheet children (table 3.7). When cover-sheet children are included, Medicaid coverage of the poor increased 6 percentage points between 1988 and 1991 (table 3.8). The increase in Medicaid coverage partly reflects the federally mandated eligibility expansions. It also reflects the growth in the number of persons enrolled in AFDC. Even with the gains in Medicaid coverage, though, Medicaid still covers less than half of the poor, whether or not cover-sheet children are included.

Although not so dramatic, Medicaid coverage of the near-poor, those with incomes between 100 percent and 200 percent of poverty, has been steadily rising since the mid-1980s. These gains reflect the impact of the eligibility expansions.

Despite expanding Medicaid coverage, the proportion of the population without health insurance has recently been growing. From 1988 to 1991, uninsurance rates increased from 13.4 percent to 14.1 percent, including cover-sheet children (table 3.8). In percentage

Table 3.7 PERCENTAGE DISTRIBUTION OF U.S. POPULATION BY TYPE OF HEALTH CARE INSURANCE COVERAGE
(HIERARCHICAL), Excluding Cover-Sheet Children: 1984–91

Total Population (Poor, near-poor, nonpoor)

	Year[a]						
	1984	1986	1988	1989	1990	1991
Population (000s)	243,020	238,744	243,685	246,191	248,886	251,394
Hierarchical Level[b]	100%	100%	100%	100%	100%	100%
Medicaid	8.3	8.3	8.0	8.0	9.0	9.7
Employer	56.7	57.2	60.5	60.0	58.7	58.0
Other public[c]	12.0	12.1	9.8	9.7	9.6	9.6
Own private	7.1	6.6	6.7	6.8	6.8	6.5
Uninsured[d]	16.0	15.8	15.1	15.5	15.9	16.1

Poor (up to 100 percent of federal poverty line)

	Year[a]						
	1984	1986	1988	1989	1990	1991
Population (000s)	35,563	34,263	33,502	33,336	35,782	37,694
Hierarchical Level[b]	100%	100%	100%	100%	100%	100%
Medicaid	39.4	40.4	39.6	39.6	42.2	44.2
Employer	11.5	9.5	10.1	10.5	9.0	8.3
Other public[c]	8.1	8.9	9.1	8.7	9.4	8.4
Own private	7.1	6.6	6.9	6.5	6.1	5.8
Uninsured[d]	33.9	34.6	34.3	34.7	33.2	33.4

Near Poor (between 100 percent and 200 percent of federal poverty line)

	Year[a]					
	1984	1986	1988	1989	1990	1991
Population (000s)	47,024	45,097	45,256	45,561	46,604	48,489
Hierarchical Level[b]	100%	100%	100%	100%	100%	100%
Medicaid	8.0	8.7	9.1	9.2	10.2	11.0
Employer	40.6	39.8	40.3	38.9	39.0	39.1
Other public[c]	19.1	19.4	18.0	18.3	16.7	17.3
Own private	8.7	7.8	7.8	7.6	7.4	6.4
Uninsured	23.6	24.4	24.8	26.0	26.6	26.3

Sources: Current Population Surveys of U.S. Bureau of the Census, edited by the Urban Institute's TRIM2 model.

a. Years are data years rather than survey years.

b. Persons reporting more than one type of coverage are shown in the first appropriate category. For example, a person reporting both Medicaid and employer coverage would fall into the Medicaid category.

c. Persons covered by Medicare, CHAMPUS, VA, and military health.

d. Persons who were uninsured throughout the entire year.

Table 3.8 PERCENTAGE DISTRIBUTION OF U.S. POPULATION BY TYPE OF
HEALTH CARE INSURANCE COVERAGE (HIERARCHICAL), Including
Cover-Sheet Children: 1988–91

Total Population (poor, near-poor, nonpoor)

	Year[a]			
	1988	1989	1990	1991
Population (000s)	243,685	246,191	248,886	251,394
Hierarchical Level[b]	100%	100%	100%	100%
Medicaid	8.5	8.6	9.7	10.7
Employer	61.0	60.6	59.2	58.5
Other public[c]	9.7	9.7	9.5	9.5
Own private	7.3	7.6	7.5	7.2
Uninsured[d]	13.4	13.6	13.9	14.1

Poor (up to 100 percent of federal poverty line)

	Year[a]			
	1988	1989	1990	1991
Population (000s)	33,502	33,336	35,782	37,694
Hierarchical Level[b]	100%	100%	100%	100%
Medicaid	41.2	41.9	44.9	47.3
Employer	11.2	11.6	10.2	9.1
Other public[c]	9.0	8.5	9.1	8.3
Own private	7.8	7.4	7.1	6.7
Uninsured[d]	30.8	30.5	28.7	28.6

Near Poor (between 100 percent and 200 percent of federal poverty line)

	Year[a]			
	1988	1989	1990	1991
Population (000s)	45,256	45,561	46,604	48,489
Hierarchical Level[b]	100%	100%	100%	100%
Medicaid	9.9	10.1	11.4	12.4
Employer	41.2	40.0	39.8	39.8
Other public[c]	18.0	18.2	16.7	17.2
Own private	8.7	8.7	8.3	7.2
Uninsured[d]	22.2	23.0	23.8	23.4

Sources: Current Population Surveys of U.S. Bureau of the Census, edited by the
Urban Institute's TRIM2 model.
a. Years are data years rather than survey years.
b. Persons reporting more than one type of coverage are shown in the first appropriate
category. For example, a person reporting both Medicaid and employer coverage would
fall into the Medicaid category.
c. Persons covered by Medicare, CHAMPUS, VA, and military health.
d. Persons who were uninsured throughout the entire year.

terms this increase seems relatively minor, but when translated into number of persons, the growth in the uninsured is compelling: between 1988 and 1991, the number of people without health insurance increased by more than 2.8 million, including cover-sheet children.[8] Although the proportion of the population lacking health insurance has grown in recent years, over the longer term, uninsurance rates have been relatively stable. In 1991, 16.1 percent of the population was uninsured (excluding cover-sheet children), up only slightly from 16 percent in 1984 (table 3.7).

Some of the recent increase in the number of people without health care coverage can be attributed to declining employment-based health care coverage. Including cover-sheet children, the proportion of the total population with employment-related coverage decreased from 61 percent in 1988 to 58.5 percent in 1991 (table 3.8). This erosion of employer-based coverage was observed regardless of income. Eroding employment-based health care coverage could have been caused by the recent recession—in which many people lost jobs that provided health insurance—or by employers deciding to terminate health care benefits because of rising insurance costs. Another factor may be the continuing economywide shift from industries that are likely to provide insurance (such as manufacturing) to those that are not (such as the service sector).

Although overall the share of the population without health care protection has been rising, among the poor, uninsurance rates have declined. When cover-sheet children are included, the poor uninsured decreased from 30.8 percent to 28.6 percent in 1991 (table 3.8). Thus, for the poor, Medicaid expanded more rapidly than the decline in employment-based coverage, causing the level of uninsurance to fall. By contrast, for the near-poor and the nonpoor, uninsurance levels rose, since employer-based insurance fell faster than Medicaid expanded.

HEALTH INSURANCE COVERAGE BY SELECT POPULATION GROUPS

Children

Medicaid coverage of children aged 18 and under has increased significantly in recent years, as seen in figure 3.1. Since 1988 the proportion of children covered by the program climbed 5 percentage

Figure 3.1 CHANGES IN HEALTH INSURANCE PATTERNS FOR CHILDREN AND ADULT WOMEN: 1988—91

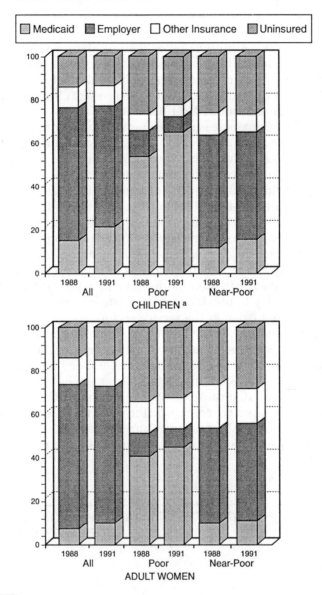

Source: Current Population Survey, U.S. Bureau of the Census.
Notes: Poor = under 100 percent of poverty; Near-Poor = 100–200 percent of poverty.
a. Includes data on "cover-sheet children."

points, so that in 1991 more than one-fifth of all children were protected by Medicaid. The growth in Medicaid coverage has been particularly steep among children living in poverty, rising nearly 10 percentage points from 1988 to 1991—from 54.3 percent to 63.6 percent. Much of this increase stems from the Medicaid eligibility expansions. Despite these large gains, though, more than 20 percent of all poor children were uninsured in 1991. However, more of these children will become eligible for Medicaid in coming years as the mandates continue to be phased in.

Reflecting the numerous Medicaid expansions targeted at children living in poverty, the proportion of poor children who lacked health insurance has substantially diminished in recent years, decreasing from 26.5 percent in 1988 to 21.3 percent in 1991 (see figure 3.1). By contrast, near-poor and nonpoor children (not shown) showed increasing rates of uninsurance between 1988 and 1991.

Adult Women

Among adult women, the share covered by Medicaid has also increased, rising from 7.5 percent to 9.2 percent over the 1988–91 time period (figure 3.1). Similar to children, the growth was greatest among poor women: the proportion covered by Medicaid rose from 40.7 percent in 1988 to 44.9 percent in 1991. Coverage of the near-poor also increased, though by not as much. These increases partly reflect the eligibility expansions, particularly those targeted at pregnant women. Some of the increases also reflect growth in number of people enrolled in the AFDC program.

Noninstitutionalized Aged

Increases in Medicaid coverage were also observed among persons aged 65 and older who did not reside in an institution (figure 3.2). In 1991 the proportion of noninstitutionalized elderly covered by Medicaid was 9.5 percent, up from 8.5 percent in 1988. This growth in Medicaid protection stems partly from the QMB mandates. Unlike children and adult women, among those aged persons living in the community, Medicaid coverage increased more rapidly for the near-poor than for the poor.

Compared to other groups, the elderly population has a very low rate of uninsurance, about 1 percent. This reflects the fact that the Medicare program covers virtually all the elderly, regardless of

Figure 3.2 CHANGES IN HEALTH INSURANCE PATTERNS FOR
NONINSTITUTIONALIZED AGED AND DISABLED ADULTS: 1988–91

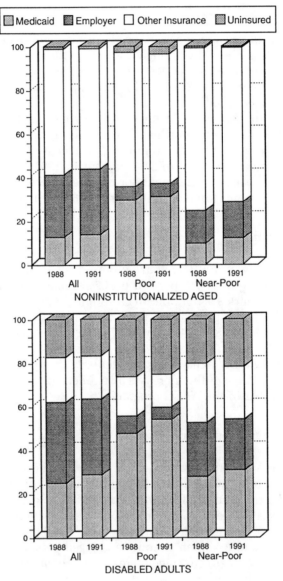

Source: Current Population Survey, U.S. Bureau of the Census.
Notes: Poor = under 100 percent of poverty; Near-Poor = 100—200 percent of poverty.

income. Although only a small fraction of the elderly lack any health care coverage, virtually all lack coverage for long-term care, since Medicare covers only acute care. In other words, although most elderly people are at risk of needing long-term care, only a very small proportion of the population has insurance coverage for these vital services.[9]

Disabled Adults

Medicaid coverage of disabled adults (those who had a health or physical disability that prevented or limited them from working) increased by more than 4 percentage points between 1988 and 1991 (figure 3.2). Among the poor disabled, the increase was still greater, growing 6.6 percentage points. By 1991, nearly 55 percent of poor disabled persons were covered by Medicaid. On the whole, the level of uninsurance among the disabled population was stable (17 percent), but a decline was observed among the poor disabled. Even with the increase in Medicaid coverage coupled with the declining uninsurance rates, nearly one-quarter of the poor disabled lacked health care insurance in 1991. (One reason for this low coverage rate may be that the definition of *disability* used by the CPS is not as restrictive as that used by the Social Security Administration in determining eligibility for SSI.)

SUMMARY

AFDC eligibility standards declined by more than 16 percent between 1980 and 1992. By 1992, the average benefit standard as a percentage of poverty was 46 percent. Thus, families had to be poorer to qualify for AFDC in 1992 than in 1980. Variation among states' benefit levels did not change much over the 1980–92 period, so inequities in AFDC families' access to Medicaid remain high across the nation.

Medically needy standards also eroded. In 1992, after adjusting for inflation, the average state's standard was $654, down from $849 in 1980. By contrast, SSI/SSP standards have generally kept pace with inflation. This reflects the fact that SSI income standards are set nationally, unlike AFDC and medically needy eligibility thresholds.

In response to growing concerns about infant mortality and eroding health care coverage of children, Congress enacted a series of legislated mandates and options expanding Medicaid to these and other populations. States generally supported these legislative actions and rapidly implemented them, particularly those targeted at pregnant women. For pregnant women and children, the expansions changed Medicaid law so that coverage for these populations is now based on income relative to the federal poverty line rather than to each state's AFDC standards, breaking the historically strong tie between AFDC and Medicaid. For pregnant women and children, there is now a set minimum income standard for Medicaid, similar to that for SSI recipients. Some of the eligibility inequities among states were corrected by these mandates.

Reflecting the eligibility expansions, the proportion of the population with Medicaid coverage has expanded rapidly in recent years: CPS data indicate that nearly 11 percent of the population was protected by Medicaid in 1991, up from 8.5 percent in 1988. Among poor people, Medicaid coverage rose from 41.2 percent to 47.3 percent during the period. However, although Medicaid rapidly expanded, less than half of the poor were covered by the program in 1991.

Even though CPS data show that Medicaid coverage greatly expanded between 1988 and 1991, the percentage of uninsured people grew slightly, from 13.4 percent to 14.1 percent for the total population. This was primarily because employer-based coverage declined more rapidly than Medicaid grew. For poor families, who are most aided by Medicaid, the proportion of uninsured fell slightly. But for the near-poor and nonpoor, uninsurance became a more severe problem.

Notes

1. Of all issues related to Medicaid, eligibility is perhaps the most complex. States, under broad federal guidelines, are allowed considerable flexibility in designing their programs and setting eligibility standards. One consequence of this flexibility is that, across the states, over 50 distinct populations are eligible for Medicaid. Thus, there are many exceptions to the general rules. Here we focus only on the major populations and eligibility trends. For a more comprehensive treatment of the subject, readers are referred elsewhere (Congressional Research Service 1993; Committee on Ways and Means 1992.

2. The coefficient of variation is the standard deviation of the benefit level divided by the mean benefit level. A coefficient of variation equal to 0 percent indicates that there is no variation; that is, all states have the same benefit level. A coefficient of

variation of 50 percent, by contrast, indicates that about 33 percent of the states have benefit levels less than half the average level or, alternatively, more than 150 percent of the average.

3. More specifically, the *Zebley* ruling required that a child's functional status must also be assessed when determining SSI eligibility. Previously, for both children and adults, an applicant's condition was compared to a list of SSI qualifying impairments. If a child did not meet the specified impairment level, he or she was determined ineligible for benefits. By contrast, if an adult did not meet the specified impairment level, an individual functional assessment would be conducted and the applicant would be reevaluated. The *Zebley* case ruled that children were also entitled to such individual assessments.

4. This option was included as part of the Omnibus Budget Reconciliation Act of 1986.

5. The CPS is performed each year on a nationally representative sample of the noninstitutionalized U.S. population. About 60,000 households participate in the survey. In addition to questions about demographics, household composition, income, and disability status, the CPS contains detailed information on respondents' health insurance coverage during the preceding year.

6. For a fuller discussion of these survey changes, readers are referred to Kronick (1991) and Levit, Olin, and Letsch (1992).

7. Multiple insurance sources may occur because a person first has one insurance type, then later has another, or because a person has two insurers at the same time.

8. In addition, the CPS underestimates the problem of uninsurance, since it counts only those who were without medical care coverage the entire year. Consequently, persons who have insurance for some part of the year but are uninsured the rest of the year would be counted as having coverage.

9. Medicaid, of course, will provide long-term care but only when impoverishment occurs. Thus Medicaid, at some level, may be viewed as long-term care insurance.

Chapter Four

EQUITY ACROSS STATES

Previous chapters of this volume have discussed recent trends in Medicaid, particularly program enrollment and expenditures nation-wide. This chapter examines distributional changes among the states. It asks: Did Medicaid coverage become more equitable across the states in the past decade? And did expenditures per recipient become more similar?

From Medicaid's inception, states have controlled critical aspects of program design, including eligibility, services, and reimbursement levels. Patterned after the earlier Kerr-Mills programs, Medicaid was built on a foundation of joint federal-state responsibility and shared financing. A longstanding and deeply rooted criticism of Medicaid is that there is substantial inequity among states: equally poor people in different states face widely disparate eligibility criteria and, once eligible for services, may receive very different care (e.g., Davis and Schoen 1978; Erdman and Wolfe 1987; Reinhardt 1985). The inequal-ity of access to Medicaid services has long been a common argument in favor of a national health insurance program.

As originally designed, Medicaid recognized that states had differ-ing fiscal resources and sought to level the playing field between rich and poor states by basing the federal match rate on per capita income in each state. Despite this, earlier analyses demonstrated that richer states still managed to have more generous programs and to draw down more federal matching funds than poor states (Holahan and Cohen 1986).

REASONS STATES MAY HAVE BECOME MORE SIMILAR

Beginning in the late 1980s, various changes occurred that may have made Medicaid more uniform across the nation. Some of these were the result of explicit federal policy decisions to make Medicaid more uniform. As described in the previous chapter, Medicaid eligibility for adults and children has been historically tied to AFDC eligibility standards, which vary greatly across states. A series of federal laws passed in the late 1980s made Medicaid eligibility more uniform for key groups, by linking program eligibility to federal poverty guidelines—especially the mandates for pregnant women and children and for qualified Medicare beneficiaries (QMBs)—instead of welfare guidelines. However, as noted in chapter 3, AFDC and medically needy income standards were declining in real terms and were not becoming more similar across states.

Other policies that began in the 1980s had the potential to equalize services and expenditures for the program. For example, OBRA 87 upgraded quality standards for nursing homes in areas such as certification and staffing, which could decrease interstate differences in service quality and cost. Likewise, the QMB provisions could standardize many aspects of program service by guaranteeing that elderly persons across the nation have comparable access to Medicare services and providers. In addition, fear of Boren Amendment lawsuits may have reduced states' abilities to modify hospital and nursing home payment rates, which could reduce the potential for interstate differences. In addition, there were gradual reforms in Medicaid operations, such as implementation of prospective payment systems for hospitals and physicians, that may have made programs more similar. Some have contended that state Medicaid programs were converging over time, that is, that the reforms were making state policies more similar (Bachman, Beatrice, and Altman 1987).

Beyond direct Medicaid policy changes, other broader forces may have served to equalize Medicaid across states. General state budgetary pressures may have led wealthier states to shrink their programs while poorer states were expanding theirs, partly influenced by the mandates. Fiscal stresses in the late 1980s and early 1990s induced many states to impose more limits on optional services and eligibility groups. States with more generous Medicaid programs, such as those in the Northeast, had more that could be cut, whereas states with few optional services or eligibility groups had less ability to cut. Simultaneously, the disproportionate-share (DSH) and special financing programs (provider taxes and donations programs) may have reduced interstate differences, since poorer states with high federal matching rates had greater incentives to develop these programs. Thus, regional economic forces may have interacted with Medicaid policies to equalize the program in the past decade.

EQUITY OF MEDICAID PROGRAM COVERAGE

The equity of Medicaid services is measured in two dimensions: (1) *program coverage*, which examines the ratio of Medicaid recipients in each state to a broader population measure such as the number of people in poverty or the number of elderly persons and (2) *expenditures per recipient*, which represents average Medicaid expenditures per recipient in each state.[1] Both dimensions combine a number of different aspects of Medicaid. Program coverage is affected primarily by a state's eligibility criteria, but is also somewhat affected by utilization of services. In general, 80 percent to 90 percent of those enrolled in Medicaid actually use any medical services in a given year. Program expenditures per recipient are affected by the range, type, and limitations of services available to recipients, as well as by reimbursement levels paid to providers.

The statistic used to measure equity among the states is the unweighted *coefficient of variation*, the standard deviation of a variable divided by its mean. We also report the *weighted mean*, in which states are counted proportionate to their size, and the *unweighted mean*, in which all states are counted equally.

Table 4.1 presents the ratio of Medicaid recipients (persons actually receiving service) to persons under 100 percent of poverty in each state in 1979, 1984, 1989, and 1991. This is a good general measure of the relative size of Medicaid programs, although some persons with incomes above poverty are eligible for Medicaid.[2] Data on persons in poverty are best for 1979 and 1989, since these data come from the 1980 and 1990 Censuses of the Population, respectively. The 1984 and 1991 poverty data are from the Current Population Survey (CPS), which is a sample survey. CPS poverty estimates have relatively large standard errors for small states (U.S. Bureau of the Census 1992); thus, the 1984 and 1991 estimates are useful for examining trends, but are less reliable. Two main findings can be drawn from table 4.1:

1. Relative to the poverty population, Medicaid coverage fell substantially between 1979 and 1984, but rose in 1989 and 1991. The decline in 1984 is consistent with cutbacks made in the early 1980s that especially affected AFDC participants. By 1991, the average ratio of Medicaid recipients to poor persons was 76 percent, slightly higher than the 1979 level.
2. Access to Medicaid coverage became much more equitable across states during the decade. The coefficients of variation consistently

Table 4.1 RATIO OF MEDICAID RECIPIENTS TO PERSONS IN POVERTY,
SELECTED YEARS

State	Recipients per Person in Poverty			
	1979 (%)	1984 (%)	1989 (%)	1991 (%)
Massachusetts	157	93	111	102
Rhode Island	131	95	112	165
California	128	102	95	83
Hawaii	120	98	96	98
Pennsylvania	115	61	95	95
Maine	111	75	95	88
Wisconsin	106	67	79	84
New York	103	78	99	90
New Jersey	96	70	92	80
Michigan	95	67	85	85
Connecticut	91	101	105	98
Vermont	83	82	99	97
Illinois	83	60	79	72
Oregon	82	43	62	66
Minnesota	81	89	81	74
Ohio	75	69	86	87
Maryland	73	91	83	84
West Virginia	72	49	70	87
Washington	69	68	84	107
Oklahoma	65	57	50	56
Delaware	65	72	73	95
Kansas	65	60	63	64
Kentucky	65	64	62	76
Iowa	59	52	73	96
New Hampshire	58	59	52	73
Missouri	58	50	61	67
Colorado	53	69	51	64
Louisiana	51	43	54	81
Virginia	51	54	56	73
South Carolina	50	44	53	64
Arkansas	50	35	55	67
Mississippi	47	48	64	74
North Carolina	46	40	59	69
Alabama	46	45	44	51
Georgia	45	47	63	68
Utah	45	41	48	57
Montana	44	45	46	49
Tennessee	44	43	73	94
Indiana	44	41	54	48
Nebraska	42	41	64	85
Alaska	42	48	76	83
New Mexico	38	30	37	46
North Dakota	36	33	52	56
Idaho	35	21	36	49

(continued)

Table 4.1 RATIO OF MEDICAID RECIPIENTS TO PERSONS IN POVERTY,
SELECTED YEARS (continued)

State	Recipients per Person in Poverty			
	1979 (%)	1984 (%)	1989 (%)	1991 (%)
Florida	34	34	55	60
Texas	33	30	39	58
Nevada	32	29	37	42
South Dakota	31	33	42	60
Wyoming	31	33	54	78
Weighted mean	74	60	71	76
Unweighted mean	67	57	68	76
Coefficient of variation	45	37	30	27

Sources: Recipients are from HCFA-2082 data. For the years 1979 and 1989, data for persons in poverty are from the Census of Population. For the years 1984 and 1991, data for persons in poverty are from the Current Population Survey.
Note: Excludes Washington, D.C., Arizona, and U.S. territories.

fell between 1979 and 1991. The coefficient of variation fell by roughly half between 1979 and 1991. The first phase of change, which occurred between 1979 and 1984, was largely caused by cutbacks in generous programs, prompted by OBRA 81. The second phase, from 1984 to 1991, was mainly caused by increases in restrictive states, occasioned by the eligibility expansions for pregnant women and children.

The overall policy goals of increasing Medicaid coverage and reducing interstate differences were largely successful. Convergence occurred both as a result of retractions among the high-coverage states, as well as expansion in the low-coverage states. For the top 10 states in 1979, Medicaid recipients averaged 116 percent of the poverty population; the top 10 states in 1991 averaged 102 percent of poverty.[3] The bottom 10 states rose from an average of 35 percent in 1979 to 51 percent in 1991. Nonetheless, there was a fair degree of consistency in the relative generosity of many states over the decade. Four states consistently had higher coverage rates: Massachusetts, Rhode Island, New York, and Hawaii were among the 10 highest states in each of the years measured. Likewise, 4 states were consistently among the 10 lowest states: Nevada, Texas, New Mexico, and Idaho.

Table 4.2 presents summaries of similar analyses for Medicaid coverage in 1984 and 1991 broken down for the four eligibility groups: children, adults, aged, and blind and disabled.[4] Because reliable

Table 4.2 SUMMARY MEASURES OF MEDICAID COVERAGE AMONG STATES: 1984 AND 1991

Program Coverage	1984 (%)	1991 (%)
Ratio of Child Recipients to Population under 18 Years Old		
Weighted mean	15.3	20.2
Unweighted mean	13.4	18.9
Coefficient of variation	47.5	32.4
Ratio of Adult Recipients to Population 18 to 65 Years Old		
Weighted mean	3.3	4.2
Unweighted mean	3.0	3.9
Coefficient of variation	39.8	30.2
Ratio of Aged Recipients to Elderly Population (65 or older)		
Weighted mean	11.1	10.7
Unweighted mean	10.7	10.7
Coefficient of variation	39.9	35.4
Ratio of Blind and Disabled Recipients to Severely Disabled Population 16 to 64 Years Old		
Weighted mean	43.6	60.6
Unweighted mean	40.2	58.3
Coefficient of variation	30.9	26.9

Note: Excludes Arizona and U.S. territories.

estimates of the number of poor people by age or disability group are not available for these years, the denominators are for all people in a category without regard to income. Although this is not optimal, the inability to factor in poverty causes little, if any, bias. On the national level, poverty levels for 1984 and 1991 were almost identical.[5]

As seen in table 4.2, between 1984 and 1992, Medicaid both covered a greater share of children and adults and became more equitable across states. For children, the coefficient of variation fell about one-third, dropping from 48 percent in 1984 to 32 percent in 1991. By 1991, 20 percent of all U.S. children received Medicaid services during the year. For adults, the coefficient of variation fell about one-quarter, decreasing from 40 percent to 30 percent. The share of all adults in Medicaid rose from 3.3 percent to 4.2 percent. These gains in coverage and in equity for children and adults occurred even though AFDC and medically needy income standards were declining during the 1980s and were not converging. This indicates that the AFDC and medically needy income levels were becoming relatively less influential in affecting Medicaid caseload levels.

In comparison, there were small reductions in interstate variation among the elderly between 1984 and 1991. There was no appreciable change in the proportion of the elderly receiving Medicaid services between 1984 and 1991, and only a small reduction in interstate variation. The lack of change in coverage for the elderly is somewhat surprising, given the expansion of policies such as QMB status. It is plausible that much of the growth in this category came at the expense of other eligibility categories for the elderly, so that there was little net growth.

Medicaid provides a substantial and increasing level of care for the blind and disabled.[6] The program coverage statistics were quite high (44 percent in 1984 and 61 percent in 1991), particularly considering that income is not factored into the denominator. This growth in coverage parallels increasing participation levels of the blind and disabled in SSI, which grew 46 percent between 1984 and 1991 (Committee on Ways and Means 1992). However, the rate of adults with a self-reported severe work disability fell slightly between 1980 and 1990 (LaPlante 1993), continuing a downward trend from the peak in the 1970s (Wolfe and Haveman 1990). One possible reason for this anomaly is that changes in SSI eligibility rules, especially for children, were implemented during the period, such as the expanded eligibility of disabled children due to the 1990 Supreme Court decision in *Sullivan v. Zebley*, 1990. However, the eligibility determinations for the *Zebley* case were only partially implemented by 1991, so it cannot fully explain the increasing coverage of the disabled population in SSI. Another possible factor was the increase in AIDS cases during this time period. While this factor should have increased the actual number of disabled persons, it is possible that the self-reported work disability questions do not measure these changes very well. This increase may also have been caused by heightened awareness of and incentives for participation in SSI and Medicaid during the decade. As health care costs rose and it became more difficult to get private insurance for the disabled, there were greater incentives for the disabled (or their families) to join Medicaid. Also, providers of care to disabled persons (i.e., mental retardation or mental health institutions, including state-owned facilities) had stronger incentives to help patients enroll in SSI to get Medicaid funds as state funds became more scarce.

Coverage for the blind and disabled had less variation than the other groups. This is because eligibility for the blind and disabled, tied to SSI, is more uniform than eligibility for other groups, such as those eligible through AFDC participation. Although there is some state variation in eligibility for the disabled in Medicaid, it is much less than for other groups. While the elderly also have more similar eligibility (through SSI, QMB, and the "300 percent" rule), the incentives for the aged to join Medicaid are much smaller, since they have Medicare, Social Security, and pensions.

EQUITY OF PROGRAM EXPENDITURES PER RECIPIENT

Once people are enrolled in Medicaid, there are also differences in the type and levels of services available to them and the payments made to health care providers on their behalf. For example, a recent study found substantial variation in Medicaid physician fees when compared to localized fees for Medicare or private insurance (Holahan 1991). In that study, the Medicaid-to-Medicare or Medicaid-to-private fee ratios generally had coefficients of variation in the range of 24–27 percent.

As seen in table 4.3, expenditures per recipient vary just about as much as program coverage. States with generous eligibility are not always those with generous spending per recipient. For example, California generally tends to have higher coverage but lower expenditures per recipient, while New Hampshire tends to have lower coverage but higher expenditures per recipient.

There were essentially no changes in the interstate variation in Medicaid expenditures per adult and child recipient between 1984 and 1991. Since services to these populations involve very little long-term care, this indicates no changes in the variation of the relative spending for acute care medical services among the states. The lack of convergence is somewhat surprising. We expected that increased use of DSH payments would equalize poorer and richer states.

Although the overall variation among states did not fall, individual state rankings changed considerably. For example, only two states—Massachusetts and Maryland—and the District of Columbia were consistently in the top 10 for expenditures per adult recipient and per child recipient for both 1984 and 1991. Only one state, West Virginia, was consistently ranked in the bottom 10 for both measures for both years.

For the aged and disabled, there were small reductions in the variation in expenditures per recipient between 1984 and 1991. The slight improvements in equity are attributable to reductions in variation of expenditures per recipients for acute care, not long-term care.

Table 4.3 SUMMARY MEASURES OF MEDICAID EXPENDITURES PER
RECIPIENT IN CATEGORY AMONG STATES: 1984 AND 1991
(CONSTANT 1991 DOLLARS)

Expenditures per Recipient	1984	1991
Child—Total		
Weighted mean	$712	$1,084
Unweighted mean	$725	$1,116
Coefficient of Variation	30.9%	29.1%
Adult—Total		
Weighted mean	$1,370	$1,839
Unweighted mean	$1,371	$1,863
Coefficient of variation	24.7%	27.0%
Aged—Total		
Weighted mean	$6,195	$8,525
Unweighted mean	$6,490	$8,683
Coefficient of variation	40.9%	37.5%
Aged—Long-term care		
Weighted mean	$4,549	$6,291
Unweighted mean	$4,967	$6,471
Coefficient of variation	44.5%	44.9%
Aged—Acute Care		
Weighted mean	$1,646	$2,229
Unweighted mean	$1,521	$2,170
Coefficient of variation	47.9%	35.3%
Blind and Disabled—Total		
Weighted mean	$6,159	$7,897
Unweighted mean	$6,803	$8,597
Coefficient of variation	38.2%	36.3%
Blind and Disabled—Long-term Care		
Weighted mean	$3,195	$3,488
Unweighted mean	$3,716	$4,153
Coefficient of variation	50.0%	52.7%
Blind and Disabled—Acute Care		
Weighted mean	$2,961	$4,407
Unweighted mean	$3,087	$4,433
Coefficient of variation	42.2%	36.7%

Note: Excludes Arizona and U.S. territories.

For the elderly, the coefficient of variation fell by about one-third, from 48 percent to 35 percent between 1984 and 1991 (table 4.3).[7] It seems plausible that this is an effect of QMBs and other dually enrolled Medicaid-Medicare elderly. As Medicaid shifted from primary coverage to wraparound coverage for Medicare, there has been less interstate variation in acute care spending. There was a small decline in variation for acute care spending for the blind and disabled, but it is not clear why this occurred.

Spending per recipient for long-term care was much more variable than for acute care spending for both the aged and disabled. There are probably two main reasons for this. First, nursing home payment rates vary greatly. Analyzing the Medicaid skilled nursing facility per diem rates for 34 states in 1989, the coefficient of variation was 39 percent (data from National Governors Association 1989). Second, other policy differences may affect utilization. For example, interstate differences in eligibility for medically needy or "300 percent rule" elderly affects entry into nursing homes as well as the extent to which Medicaid or the individual pays for services. Similarly, many of the long-term care services (ICFs/MR, home and community-based care, etc.) are optional. Thus, service expenditures and utilization may vary highly for blind and disabled recipients.

Four states—Minnesota, New York, Connecticut, and Alaska—and the District of Columbia were consistently among the highest 10 for total expenditures per aged recipient and per blind or disabled recipient in 1984 and 1991. Seven states were consistently in the lowest 10: Mississippi, Alabama, California, Tennessee, Georgia, Kentucky, and Arkansas.

Differences in expenditures per recipient across states have many causes, including geographic price differences, different utilization patterns, and different service coverage and payment rates. We attempted to factor out underlying variation in health care prices using a recently developed input price index (Welch 1992).[8] After adjusting by the input price index, there was little reduction in variation. For example, the coefficient of variation for adult expenditures per recipient fell from 27.0 percent before adjustment to 25.8 percent after adjustment. Relatively little of the variation in Medicaid expenditures per recipient is caused by underlying price differences.

SUMMARY

This chapter's main finding is that Medicaid program coverage, measured relative to the poverty population, became substantially more similar across states between 1979 and 1991. Between 1979 and 1984, interstate differences shrank as more generous states trimmed Medicaid eligibility in response to OBRA 81 and the recession of that period. Nationwide, coverage declined during that time. Between 1984 and 1991, equalization occurred as less-generous states increased coverage, largely in response to federal mandates for pregnant women and children. In general, program coverage grew between 1984 and 1991. Although Medicaid coverage is still highly uneven across the nation, interstate differences fell by almost half over the past decade.

In contrast, there were few measures by which expenditures per recipient became more similar. Despite policy changes such as DSH payments, the Boren Amendment, and the OBRA 87 nursing home quality standards, states remained quite dissimilar in their average expenditures per recipient. There were declines in the variation in acute care spending for the elderly, probably as an effect of QMBs and other dually enrolled Medicaid-Medicare aged. Variation in acute care spending for the blind and disabled fell somewhat, although the reason is not clear.

Even if Medicaid was nationally uniform, interstate differences would persist because of underlying variations in the health status of populations, availability of health care providers, differences in utilization patterns, and geographic prices for health care. We can obtain a rough assessment of variation in a nationally uniform program by examining Medicare. Since Medicare rules, coverage, and structures are quite different from Medicaid, the comparisons only provide crude benchmarks. For 1989 the coefficient of variation for the proportion of Medicare recipients to enrollees was 6.7 percent and for Medicare reimbursements per recipient was 15.9 percent (based on data from Committee on Ways and Means 1992). Since almost all persons over 65 years of age are enrolled in Medicare, the ratio of recipients to enrollees approximates the ratio of recipients to the aged population. By this standard, Medicaid coverage for various groups had roughly four to five times the variation seen in Medicare, and Medicaid acute care expenditures per recipient had roughly twice the variation seen in Medicare. Although interstate differences in coverage and expenditures can never be completely eliminated, Medicaid is far less uniform than Medicare, and the differences in coverage are particularly sharp. Although states' Medicaid coverage became much more similar over the past decade, Medicaid eligibility policies are still far from attaining a level of uniformity comparable to Medicare.

Notes

1. This chapter analyzes recipients or expenditures per recipient, since there are no

enrollment data for 1979. The analyses end in 1991, since poverty data for 1992 were not available. In table 4.1, the District of Columbia is excluded owing to lack of data about 1979. Arizona, Massachusetts Blind, and U.S. territories are excluded in all analyses.

2. A key difference between these analyses and the CPS analyses in chapter 3 is that the current analyses use HCFA-2082 data to estimate the number of people receiving Medicaid services, whereas chapter 3 used self-reports of Medicaid recipiency, although both use Census data to estimate the number of people in poverty. Census data are not appropriate for these state-by-state analyses, since the sample size of Medicaid recipients in the CPS is generally quite small and the decennial Census does not ask about Medicaid receipt. As discussed in chapter 3, CPS data underestimate the number of Medicaid enrollees or recipients, when compared to the HCFA-2082 data. HCFA-2082 data do not break out Medicaid recipients with incomes below poverty versus those with incomes above poverty, so these analyses include *all* Medicaid recipients, regardless of the true income. A recent analysis that used microsimulation to correct for underreporting of Medicaid enrollment in the CPS estimated that 29 percent of Medicaid enrollees had incomes above poverty (Winterbottom 1993).

3. These statistics should not be confused with data about the proportion of *poor* people on Medicaid. There are several reasons why the number of Medicaid recipients might exceed the number of poor people in a state. First, in some cases Medicaid eligibility thresholds can exceed poverty levels (e.g., for the medically needy or pregnant women and young children). Second, poverty is measured based on annual income, whereas Medicaid recipients may be eligible for just part of a year. Third, although the recipient data are supposed to be unduplicated counts, some are double counted because of a change in eligibility status. Fourth, the poverty population is based on noninstitutionalized people, whereas Medicaid recipients include institutionalized persons.

4. Annual data about the elderly and nonelderly populations are available for each state from the U.S. Bureau of the Census.

5. In 1984, 14.4 percent of the overall population was poor (21.5 percent for children, 11.7 percent for nonelderly adults, and 12.4 percent of elderly). In 1991, 14.2 percent of the overall population was poor (21.8 percent for children, 11.4 percent for nonelderly adults, and 12.4 percent for the elderly). Although there were modest increases in interstate income disparities between 1980 and 1990 (Barancik and Shapiro 1992), it is safe to infer that changes in Medicaid recipiency between 1984 and 1991 were primarily caused by changes in Medicaid policies, rather than changes in the number of poor people.

6. Data are limited for the analyses of the ratio of blind and disabled recipients to the blind and disabled population. Our estimates for the disabled population are based on self-reports of severe work disability for 16- to 64-year-olds from the 1980 and 1990 Censuses of Population and Housing, as reported by LaPlante (1993). The values for 1984 were interpolated. This is not completely consistent with eligibility criteria for the blind and disabled in Medicaid (for example, it excludes children), but it is the best available indicator of variation in state disability levels.

7. In the analyses of acute and long-term care spending, the base of recipients is recipients of any service, not of the specific service. Since these measures are compilations of multiple services, it is not possible to identify the number of persons receiving any acute or any long-term care service.

8. Welch's (1992) input price index is a weighted average of the HCFA hospital wage index and the Geographic Practice Cost Index for physicians. It was designed for use with broad medical services such as HMOs. It was aggregated to state levels and normalized to average 1.00.

Chapter Five

HOW STATES FINANCE MEDICAID GROWTH

The rising cost of Medicaid has been a highly visible problem for states. In August 1989, 49 of the nation's governors signed a letter to Congress asking for a moratorium on new Medicaid mandates. The following year the National Conference of State Legislatures made a similar request. The National Association of State Budget Officers (NASBO 1993b) recently stated that "the growth of Medicaid over the past several years constitutes the single largest budget problem for states." The high rates of Medicaid growth since the late 1980s would have been problematic in any time period, but they were especially onerous during the recent recession, when most states experienced serious fiscal stress.

This chapter considers the questions: How did rising Medicaid spending affect state budgets? How did states cope with Medicaid growth? and What was the role of special financing policies, such as provider taxes or disproportionate-share (DSH) payments? More specifically, we evaluate general state budget policies and efforts to handle the recent surge in Medicaid spending. Particular emphasis is given to special financing programs.

Before pursuing these issues, it should be recalled that the federal government pays a majority of Medicaid costs and that its share has increased in recent years. However, Medicaid trends are better understood by looking at state-level fiscal impacts. Most program design and management decisions are made at the state level; thus, states' budgetary problems have a direct effect on Medicaid policies. Despite the federal government's share of Medicaid costs, Medicaid represents a much smaller proportion of the federal budget than of state budgets. In 1992 federal Medicaid outlays were 4.9 percent of total federal outlays, whereas state-funded Medicaid expenditures comprised 11.8 percent of state general revenue expenditures—more than twice as high as the federal government's budget share. Although Medicaid is often the largest program in a state, at the federal level

Medicaid is dwarfed by Social Security and Medicare. Thus, the recent acceleration in Medicaid spending had less *relative* fiscal impact on the federal budget than on state budgets. Because almost all states require balanced budgets, sudden increases in Medicaid spending force state governments to cut spending in other sectors or to increase revenues.

MEDICAID AND STATE BUDGETS

A fundamental fiscal problem is that Medicaid expenditures have been rising faster than state revenues. Between 1981 and 1988, state general revenues (excluding intergovernmental funds) grew an annual 8.8 percent (in nominal dollars), whereas state-level Medicaid expenditures grew slightly faster, averaging 9.3 percent annually. These growth rates, however, diverged in the past few years: between 1988 and 1991 state general revenues grew 6.5 percent annually, while state-level Medicaid spending grew 18.7 percent per year.[1] The recent growth in Medicaid expenditures occurred while a recession was slowing states' revenues.

By any measure, Medicaid became a larger component of state budgets, as many other components shrank. Table 5.1 examines the shares of total state spending allocated to Medicaid and other budget functions, including elementary and secondary education, higher education, cash assistance (for example, AFDC, state SSI supplements, and general assistance), corrections, transportation, and other functions.[2] The table differentiates spending by revenue source:

1. *State general funds,* which include general revenues from broad-based taxes and which generally exclude earmarked revenues.
2. *Other state funds,* such as special taxes, fees, or tuition. These are often earmarked for special purposes. For Medicaid, this may include provider taxes and donations and intergovernmental transfers.
3. *Federal funds,* which are largely federal grants-in-aid for various programs such as federal matching funds for Medicaid.
4. *Total,* which includes the preceding three items plus funds from bonds not used in Medicaid.

Analyses of Medicaid spending have conventionally focused on total funds, but this does not fairly convey the actual burden to states

Table 5.1 DISTRIBUTION OF SHARES OF STATE BUDGETS BY FUNCTION AND FUNDING SOURCE

State Fiscal Year	Source of Funds	Total (billions of nominal $)	Medicaid (%)	Elementary and Secondary Education (%)	Higher Education (%)	Cash Assistance (%)	Corrections (%)	All Other (%)	Total (%)
1987	State general funds	212.6	8.1	34.2	15.5	5.3	5.0	31.8	100.0
	Other state funds	97.1	0.7	9.0	11.0	0.4	0.6	78.3	100.0
	Federal funds	89.7	26.0	11.5	6.4	10.3	0.1	45.6	100.0
	Total funds	405.3	10.2	22.8	12.3	5.2	3.0	46.7	100.0
1990	State general funds	264.5	9.5	33.5	14.6	4.9	5.5	32.1	100.0
	Other state funds	110.8	1.4	10.6	15.3	0.5	0.8	71.4	100.0
	Federal funds	110.9	31.8	11.5	3.2	10.4	0.1	43.0	100.0
	Total funds	496.1	12.5	22.8	12.2	5.0	3.4	44.1	100.0
1992	State general funds	289.9	11.8	34.3	13.8	5.2	5.9	29.0	100.0
	Other state funds	152.3	6.3	8.3	13.3	0.6	0.8	70.8	100.0
	Federal funds	140.4	38.6	10.2	5.2	9.4	0.1	36.5	100.0
	Total funds	595.9	17.1	21.4	11.5	5.1	3.5	41.5	100.0

Source: National Association of State Budget Officers (1993b).
Note: "Total funds" also includes funds from bonds (not shown). Includes all 50 states and Washington, D.C.

of paying for Medicaid. Between 1987 and 1992, total federal and state Medicaid spending grew from 10.2 to 17.1 percent of total state spending (table 5.1). The only other large budget function that grew was corrections, which rose from 3 percent to 3.5 percent of state spending. Total spending for all the other functions, including elementary, secondary and higher education, and other functions shrank. Cash assistance kept the same share of total spending. In nominal dollar terms, total Medicaid spending grew an average 28 percent per year between 1990 and 1992. Total expenditures are useful in measuring total programmatic activity, but do not represent the "cost" to the state, since they include federal and nonstate funds.

State general funds best reflect real state "effort" in spending; they correspond to revenues raised from state sales taxes, income taxes, and other general revenue sources. Since the general fund is not earmarked, there is great competition for these funds. When examined from the perspective of state general funds, Medicaid's share was somewhat smaller, comprising 8.1 percent in 1987 and 11.8 percent in 1992 (table 5.1). Given the controversy about use of special revenue sources, it is important to note that "regular" state-funded spending for Medicaid did actually grow substantially in recent years and was the fastest-growing component in both the 1987–90 and 1990–92 periods. Corrections also grew, but at a slower rate. Elementary and secondary education and cash assistance stayed roughly constant. Higher education and other functions lost ground. State general fund Medicaid spending (in nominal dollars) grew an average of 17 percent per year between 1990 and 1992.

To states, one of the most important effects of Medicaid growth was the surge in federal funds. By 1992, two out of every five (39 percent) federal dollars coming to states were for Medicaid. In contrast, no other budget function showed growth in the share of federal dollars. One analyst has pointed out that during most of the 1980s federal grants to states for most purposes shrank substantially; consequently, Medicaid became the main method by which states could increase federal revenues (Miller 1992). Although Medicaid growth increases state expenditures, it also brings in at least as many federal dollars (and much more in states with a federal matching rate in excess of 50 percent). A major budget strategy for states was to maximize federal Medicaid revenues. Between 1990 and 1992, the level of federal funds grew 24 percent per year.

Perhaps the most distinctive state financing trend was the ninefold increase in the use of "other state funds" for Medicaid between 1987 and 1992. The level of other state funds used for Medicaid in dollar terms soared 149 percent per year between 1990 and 1992. This largely reflects the growth of provider taxes, donations, and intergovernmental transfers, discussed in more depth later in the chapter. These funds were used to leverage higher federal funds for Medicaid. Higher education also saw increasing levels of other state funds, caused largely by increases in tuition and other fees in state universities and colleges.

It has often been said that Medicaid "crowded out" almost all other state programs because of the competition for limited state funds. This view is somewhat exaggerated, since most analyses do not account for the lopsided growth of Medicaid funds coming from federal and "other" state sources. Although total Medicaid spending grew 28 percent per year between 1990 and 1992, state general fund spending rose only 17 percent. Nonetheless, by any measure Medicaid spending has increased substantially in recent years and has had substantial consequences for state budgets. A particular complaint about the entitlement growth of Medicaid is that the increased pressure on state general funds made it much harder to fund discretionary programs and new initiatives.

The rising cost of Medicaid was not the only source of distress for state budget-makers. Unprojected Medicaid spending surges have led to some state budget crises. Some unforeseen spending increases are caused by unanticipated changes in the economy or in health care prices, but court rulings and changing federal rules have also made Medicaid unpredictable for states. Sometimes shortfalls are partly political in nature; spending projections or appropriations can be deliberately set low to ease initial budget negotiations. Regardless of the reason, Medicaid expenditures were higher than expected. In 1992 actual state-level expenditures for Medicaid (excluding federal funds and in some cases local funds) exceeded original appropriations by 6.1 percent; in 17 states the level of overspending was more than 10 percent of the Medicaid budget. Since Medicaid is a dominant portion of the budget, this means that state legislatures often had to convene emergency sessions to "fix" the problem, such as appropriating supplemental funds. In 1992, 19 states passed supplemental funding for Medicaid (NASBO 1993a).

Revenue Increases

In addition to changing shares in the state budget, states have also increased their total revenue levels to accommodate Medicaid spending growth. Although it is a political truism that tax increases are unpopular with voters, states did increase tax effort during the 1980s and 1990s. In fact, states enacted revenue increases of $10 billion in 1991 and another $15 billion in 1992 (National Governors Association and NASBO 1992). Some of these tax increases were provider taxes (discussed later in the chapter), but there were also general tax increases such as sales, personal income, or corporate income tax increases. These tax increases were used to help mend general state budget problems, as well as to fund spiraling Medicaid costs. Some states also passed special earmarked taxes to pay for health care, including Medicaid. For example, California and Florida increased cigarette taxes and earmarked revenue for health care. In addition to generating revenue, these "sin" taxes have the political appeal of linking behaviors that worsen health to expenditures for health care. It is not surprising that President Clinton also proposed using sin taxes to pay for his national health care reform proposal.

STATE EFFORTS TO CONTAIN MEDICAID COSTS

States did not sit by passively as Medicaid spending soared. On the contrary, state Medicaid agencies became increasingly active in the management of their programs to rein in cost increases. Yet, the expenditure increases discussed occurred *despite* a wide variety of cost-containment efforts initiated by states. Based on case studies of nine states, we learned that most states made numerous cost-containment changes in Medicaid between 1988 and 1992 (Holahan et al. 1992). A national survey of states has indicated similar types of changes in 1992 and 1993 (NASBO 1993a).

The most common cost-containment mechanisms involved reducing or freezing reimbursement levels for providers, including physicians, nursing homes, and hospitals. Another common mechanism involved programs to reduce or control utilization. Smaller optional services, such as podiatry, were sometimes eliminated. States also used the federal drug rebate program and other policies to contain drug price increases. Finally, many states initiated or expanded managed care programs, especially for AFDC-type clients. Although such programs sometimes did not have short-term savings (because of initial developmental costs), states hoped that they would save money and improve access in the long run. In most cases Medicaid eligibility was not cut or was cut only in modest ways. Many of these policy changes are discussed in more depth in chapters 6 and 7.

In general, states avoided draconian cuts in Medicaid. In our discussions with state officials, several major reasons were cited for Medicaid's relatively favored position in the budget. First, health care was politically popular. For example, efforts to eliminate medically needy programs in a couple of states were rebuffed after vocal protests from patients and providers. Second, many parts of Medicaid were technically off-limits because of federal mandates or court rulings, including Boren Amendment lawsuits. Third, since Medicaid earns federal dollars, it is less advantageous to cut Medicaid than state-only programs. Thus, medical assistance programs for general assistance recipients (and general assistance programs in general) often suffered major reductions or elimination. Although these state-only indigent care programs were not technically Medicaid, they were often administered alongside Medicaid and were usually established to fill perceived gaps in Medicaid. Fourth, there were other mechanisms to help the Medicaid fiscal situation, especially special revenue programs, discussed in the following section.

SHIFTING COSTS TO THE FEDERAL GOVERNMENT

Medicaid Maximization

While states cut their programs, they also sought to increase federal revenue by shifting other state health care costs into Medicaid, especially mental health, mental retardation, and maternal and child health services. Under the so-called Medicaid maximization strategy, states reconfigured state-funded programs to be compatible with Medicaid rules to earn federal matching funds. For example, as Medicaid eligibility for pregnant women and children expanded, states used less state Maternal and Child Health funding to serve these clients and replaced it with Medicaid money. Another strategy was to transfer many AIDS patients—generally single men—from general assistance programs to SSI, making them eligible for federal Medicaid dollars. On paper, these appeared to be increasing Medicaid costs, but they really cut state-level costs by earning federal matching. The incentives for shifting state-funded health care into Medicaid has always existed; conversions have been common in many states for years. However, as state fiscal stress has increased, the pressure to find savings through such conversions has become even stronger in recent years. These conversions were not just paper transfers, however. Programs usually had to be redesigned to correspond to Medicaid rules, such as entitlement status, statewide applicability, or Medicaid quality standards. At least part of the reason states delayed was due to these issues.

Unfortunately, we cannot assess the level of shifting reliably because of lack of data. Looking at the recent increases in mental health and mental retardation expenditures (see chapter 6), expenditures per enrollee rose among ICFs/MR just a little higher than the rate of inflation between 1990 and 1992, and the constant dollar growth rate actually fell during 1984–90 and 1990–92. Mental health expenditures did increase sharply between 1991 and 1992, but most of this appears to be related to disproportionate-share (DSH) spending and intragovernmental transfers, and not to Medicaid maximization. Thus, although we suspect that Medicaid maximization had some impact on Medicaid growth, it was probably not very great.

Special Financing Programs

The most important and controversial development in Medicaid in the late 1980s and early 1990s was special state financing strategies: provider taxes, provider donations, intergovernmental transfers, and DSH programs. These financing mechanisms enabled states to shift a greater share of expenditures to the federal government while increasing payments to targeted hospitals and other providers such as mental facilities and nursing homes. Critics viewed these strategies as complicated kickback schemes to raid federal coffers, whereas advocates defended them as the only way to keep Medicaid and public hospitals afloat during the tough fiscal times. From virtual nonexistence in the mid-1980s, by 1992 these special programs encompassed $17.4 billion in DSH payments and $7.7 billion in provider taxes, donations, and intergovernmental transfers.

The special revenue programs work in a variety of ways, but a simplified example is illustrative here. Before such a program is implemented, a state Medicaid program pays a hospital $1,000 for a particular procedure. Assuming a 50 percent match rate, half of the $1,000 is paid by the state and half by the federal government. Then the state implements a tax program—or donation program— requiring the hospital to pay $400 to the state. Now the state, through its disproportionate share program, pays the hospital $1,000 for the procedure plus $500 in a disproportionate share payment. The state later reports an expenditure of $1,500 to the federal government and receives a $750 federal match. In sum, the hospital's net reimbursement increases from $1,000 to $1,100, the state reduces its contribution from $500 to $350, and the federal contribution increases from $500 to $750. The reported state-funded Medicaid expenditure is $750 but the "true" or "adjusted" state expenditure is $350. By contrast, the federal government's reported and actual expenditure is $750.

In general, special financing programs use one or more of four basic revenue sources:

1. *Provider taxes.* Taxes or assessments on certain groups of providers including hospitals, nursing homes, and physicians. The taxes are most commonly levied as a proportion of provider revenue or on a per bed basis.
2. *Provider donations.* Voluntary contributions made to the state by providers, usually hospitals or local governments, on behalf of Medicaid.
3. *Intergovernmental transfers.* Transfers from local governments (counties, cities, or hospital tax districts) to the state on behalf of Medicaid. In some cases these could overlap with tax or donation programs. The transfers are usually from areas with locally funded public hospitals that have heavy caseloads of Medicaid and uncompensated care patients.
4. *Intragovernmental transfers.*[4] Transfers from one state agency to be used on behalf of Medicaid. These are used for state-owned hospitals, such as state psychiatric hospitals or state university teaching hospitals.

For these revenues to qualify for federal matching, they had to have an outlet for expenditures. The main mechanism was disproportionate-share programs. Whereas federal law permits states great flexibility in determining Medicaid hospital payment methods and levels, the payment method must be consistent across the state and cannot exceed the Medicare payment. Since 1986, federal law has allowed state Medicaid programs to make special payments that exceed the Medicare level to selected hospitals serving a disproportionate share of low-income patients such as Medicaid and charity care patients. By exploiting the special DSH payment rules, states found a way to spend money collected from special revenue programs, while targeting the money to hospitals that served needy patients. DSH payments were not necessarily linked to a regular hospital payment; they were often made in large lump-sum payments on a periodic basis. In some cases, other expenditure outlets were used, including increased payment rates to nursing homes or physicians. Regular payments to hospitals could also be increased if they did not exceed the Medicare level.

In many states DSH payments were linked to levels of uncompensated care provided by hospitals. An important effect was that state Medicaid programs were often indirectly subsidizing uncompensated care to uninsured patients. Thus, Medicaid was paying for care for substantial numbers of people not enrolled in or eligible for the program. On an anecdotal basis, hospitals used these funds in a variety of ways such as providing better care, building new clinics, and reducing debt. Since many of the DSH hospitals are public hospitals, improvements in their financial status aided local governments. On the other hand, some states appeared to have used these programs primarily to reduce their state deficits, and little of the additional money was used to fund more health care (Morgan 1993).

States often developed multiple programs that targeted different sets of providers (Health Policy Alternatives 1992; Holahan et al. 1992). The programs were generally complex and involved negotiations between Medicaid officials, providers, legislators, and attorneys. In some cases, the programs were established to help increase payments to providers in response to Boren Amendment challenges. In the early years, these programs were often designed to channel DSH expenditures back to the same hospitals that provided donations, taxes, or transfers. This has become more difficult recently. The Medicaid Voluntary Contributions and Provider-Specific Tax Amendments of 1991 set limits on these programs; most of the provisions began to be effective in 1993.[5] The legislation essentially:

☐ Bans provider donations for most reasons,
☐ Requires that provider taxes be "broad-based" taxes across an entire class of providers, such as acute care hospitals, nursing homes, and so forth, and caps the revenues at 25 percent of state Medicaid spending,
☐ Prohibits states from guaranteeing that DSH payments will exceed the tax payment for each hospital, and
☐ Permits HCFA to set state caps for DSH payments based on fiscal year 1992 DSH levels or a 12 percent national target and specifies certain rules for designating DSH hospitals.

These new rules changed the fiscal environment for states substantially for fiscal year 1993: states had to terminate donation programs, substantially revise or add tax programs, and modify their DSH programs. Further, the DSH caps effectively curtailed the potential for growth in DSH.

Special Revenue Sources: Provider Taxes, Donations, and Intergovernmental Revenues

The first provider tax program was a broad-based tax on physicians levied by Florida in 1984. But the origin of special financing mechanisms is more conventionally traced to West Virginia in 1986, when that state sought permission to use donations from hospitals and to increase payments to hospitals through the DSH program. But, as seen in table 5.2, the real growth spurt for these programs occurred in the 1991–92 period. The programs began in southeastern states and subsequently proliferated in that region. These states had the greatest incentive to develop special programs: they had high federal matching rates and had to expand to meet federal mandates of the late 1980s.

As seen in the lower panel of table 5.2, between 1991 and 1992 the revenues from provider donation programs shrank, while those from provider tax and intergovernmental transfer programs grew. Since the 1991 legislation banned provider donations, the reduced use of donation programs by 1992 is not surprising. Many of the 1992 donation and tax programs were temporary programs established for a year or less; states knew that many of these programs would be prohibited in 1993. There was extremely rapid growth in revenues from intergovernmental transfers (and intragovernmental transfers, not shown), which were not directly regulated by the 1991 legislation. The requirement that provider taxes be broad-based meant that almost any provider tax would yield both winners (those whose DSH payments exceed the tax) and losers (those whose tax payments exceed DSH payments), causing serious legislative struggles. Anecdotal information suggests that inter- and intragovernmental transfers have become even more important in 1993 (Intergovernmental Health Policy Project 1993c).

Using these data, we can net out the impact of provider taxes, donations, and intergovernmental transfers on Medicaid growth to try to get a better sense of "true" state-level spending on Medicaid. Table 5.3 presents information about Medicaid spending with and without these special revenues. Between 1988 and 1992, state-level Medicaid spending grew an average of 20.9 percent per year, but if we net out revenue from provider taxes, donations, and intergovernmental transfers, this declines to 16.0 percent per year.[6] Between

Table 5.2 REVENUES RECEIVED BY STATES FROM SPECIAL REVENUES (PROVIDER TAXES, DONATIONS, AND INTERGOVERNMENTAL TRANSFERS [IGTs]) BY DHHS REGION: 1985–92

DHHS Region	Sum of Provider Taxes, Donations, and IGTs (millions of nominal $)							
	1985	1986	1987	1988	1989	1990	1991	1992
I — New England							587.3	997.4
II — New York–New Jersey							169.7	641.2
III — Mid-Atlantic			20.0				254.0	213.7
IV — Southeast	24.1	74.5	106.6	136.1	151.0	307.3	714.1	1,663.0
V — Midwest					26.7	38.0	353.9	1,441.8
VI — South Central					6.6	35.9	437.5	764.3
VII — Plains States							236.1	511.8
VIII — Mountain States							6.1	86.8
IX — West						21.9	79.9	1,399.2
X — Pacific Northwest							42.8	79.5
Total, United States	24.1	74.5	126.6	136.1	184.3	403.2	2,881.3	7,798.7
Number of states with programs	1	1	2	2	5	6	34	39

DHHS Region	Provider Taxes		Donations		IGTs	
	1991	1992	1991	1992	1991	1992
I — New England	583.0	818.4	4.0	2.4	0.3	179.0
II — New York–New Jersey	159.5	410.9		27.9	10.2	227.9
III — Mid-Atlantic	89.0	134.3	165.0	311.4		51.5
IV — Southeast	309.6	945.6	291.0	218.4	113.5	406.1
V — Midwest	152.9	956.3	200.9	47.3		267.0
VI — South Central	354.7	376.8	72.3	201.6	10.5	340.2
VII — Plains States		0.0	196.7	10.3	39.4	310.2
VIII — Mountain States		18.4	6.1	1.6		58.1
IX — West	3.2	97.2	74.7		2.0	1,300.4
X — Pacific Northwest	36.5	35.4	6.2	37.7		6.4
Total, United States	1,688.4	3,793.3	1,017.1	858.5	175.9	3,146.9
Number of states with programs	22	29	18	23	8	28

Note: DHHS, U.S. Department of Health and Human Services. Data are compiled from various sources, including the HCFA and the National Association of Public Hospitals. Because the HCFA did not require reporting until 1992, the quality of the historical data is uncertain. In addition, data do not include estimates of intragovernmental transfers.

Table 5.3 FEDERAL AND STATE MEDICAID SPENDING GROWTH, 1988–92: INCLUDING AND EXCLUDING SPECIAL REVENUES (PROVIDER TAXES, DONATIONS, AND INTERGOVERNMENTAL TRANSFERS)

| | | Expenditure Levels (billions of nominal dollars) | | | | | |
| | Federal Spending ($) | State Spending ($) | | Total Spending ($) | | Federal Share of Total Spending (%) | |
Year		Including Special Revenues	Excluding Special Revenues	Including Special Revenues	Excluding Special Revenues	Including Special Revenues	Excluding Special Revenues
1988	28.8	22.5	22.3	51.3	51.1	56.1	56.4
1989	32.7	25.4	25.2	58.1	57.9	56.3	56.5
1990	39.0	30.0	29.6	69.0	68.6	56.5	56.9
1991	49.8	37.6	34.7	87.4	84.5	57.0	58.9
1992	64.8	48.1	40.3	112.9	105.1	57.4	61.7
Period	Average Annual Growth (nominal dollars) (%)						
1988–92	22.5	20.9	15.9	21.8	19.8		
1990–92	28.9	26.6	16.7	27.9	23.8		
1988–89	13.5	12.9	13.1	13.3	13.3		
1989–90	19.3	18.1	17.4	18.8	18.4		
1990–91	27.7	25.3	17.3	26.7	23.2		
1991–92	30.1	27.9	16.1	29.2	24.4		

Note: Data are compiled from various sources, including the HCFA and the National Association of Public Hospitals. Because the HCFA did not require reporting until 1992, the quality of the historical data is uncertain. In addition, data do not include estimates of intragovernmental transfers.

1990 and 1992, the impact was even more pronounced: 26.7 percent per year including special revenues and 16.7 percent excluding them.

Although special revenues are responsible for a large share of recent state-level Medicaid spending increases, after netting them out states were still increasing Medicaid spending about 17 percent per year between 1990 and 1992, a rapid rate of growth. This estimate of the change in actual state-level spending on Medicaid is about the same as the estimate of increased Medicaid spending from state general revenues, mentioned earlier. The "true" adjusted rate of state-level Medicaid spending in 1990–92 growth was still higher than in the years before.

States differed in the degree to which they increased use of these revenue sources. For example, Missouri's state-level spending rose 54 percent per year from 1990 to 1992 if special revenues are included, but only 18 percent per year if they are excluded. In contrast, Florida's use was more modest; its state-level spending growth was 28 percent including special revenues, but 26 percent if they are excluded.

One of the main effects of these programs was that states managed to shift program costs to the federal government by using special revenues for a "paper transfer" of funds. Table 5.3 also shows the regular and "true, adjusted" levels of the overall federal share of Medicaid expenditures. In 1992, the overall federal matching share was 57.4 percent, if special revenues are included. But when special revenues are excluded, the federal share rises to 61.6 percent and the corresponding state share falls to 38.4 percent. Note, however, that the federal share would have risen a little anyway between 1988 and 1992, because of the growth of Medicaid among poorer states and because of general shifts in the nation's income distribution (Miller 1992).

Disproportionate-Share Programs

While provider taxes, donations, and intergovernmental transfers represent the revenue side of special financing programs, DSH programs are the expenditure side. Special revenue programs and DSH programs are often linked, but one does not technically require the other. For example, a nursing home tax could be linked with increases in nursing home payments without use of DSH programs. Similarly, a state could have a DSH program using only "regular" Medicaid funds. DSH payments are authorized only for inpatient hospital and inpatient mental health care.

Table 5.4 MEDICAID DISPROPORTIONATE SHARE PAYMENTS FOR ACUTE
AND MENTAL HEALTH HOSPITALS BY DHHS REGION: 1989–92

	DHHS Region	(millions of nominal $)			
		1989	1990	1991	1992
New England	I	4.9	3.9	744.5	1,522.8
New York–New Jersey	II	141.2	35.7	1,500.0	3,878.6
Mid-Atlantic	III	27.2	13.0	445.0	1,350.3
Southeast	IV	173.2	462.4	807.6	2,529.8
Midwest	V	65.1	129.0	372.6	1,572.2
South Central	VI	84.0	129.7	389.2	2,767.4
Plains States	VII	42.4	79.3	281.7	928.6
Mountain States	VIII	3.5	5.1	4.7	306.8
West	IX	10.8	11.2	101.9	2,305.4
Pacific Northwest	X	16.6	32.4	31.9	265.3
Total, United States		568.8	901.5	4,679.0	17,427.2
Number of states with programs		39	37	40	50

Note: Data are compiled from various sources, including the HCFA and one National Association of Public Hospitals. Because the HCFA did not require reporting until 1992, the quality of the historical data is uncertain.

Table 5.4 summarizes the trends in DSH payments between 1989 and 1992. Although the growth in the payment levels parallels the growth of special revenue programs, there was a steep increase in DSH payments, particularly in 1991 and 1992. By 1992, DSH programs totaled $17.4 billion, of which the federal share was $10.1 billion. However, more states had DSH programs than had special revenue programs, especially in 1989–90. Thus, many small DSH programs did not rely on special revenue programs but used regular Medicaid appropriated funds.

On August 13, 1993, the HCFA published rules that capped allowable DSH payments for 1993 and beyond. States that had high levels of DSH payments in 1992 (greater than 12 percent of their total Medicaid expenditures) were capped at their 1992 levels. States with lower DSH payments (under 12 percent) were capped at their 1992 levels, plus an estimated "growth" amount, based on estimated overall program costs. These rules represented a compromise from an interim rule issued in November 1992 that froze all states at their 1992 levels, by permitting the "low-DSH" states to increase DSH payments in line with overall program growth.

Two more recent controversies about DSH payments were that DSH hospitals sometimes served no or very few Medicaid patients; this was primarily the case for state mental institutions in which most patients were considered uncompensated care cases. Also, sometimes DSH payments greatly exceeded the cost of caring for Medicaid and uncompensated care patients. Under legislation passed in 1993, DSH payments can only be made for hospitals with at least 1 percent Medicaid volume, and DSH payments to hospitals cannot exceed the level of unreimbursed Medicaid and charity care.

Uncertain Overall Impact of Special Financing Programs

Prior to the implementation of the 1991 law, revenues from providers were often linked to DSH payments. That is, the pool of hospitals getting DSH payments was similar, although not necessarily identical, to the pool of hospitals providing the revenue. Programs were generally designed so that most participating hospitals would gain or at least break even, that is, so that the DSH payments equaled or exceeded their contributions. A hospital's *direct gain* from a program could be computed as the difference of the DSH payments (or other increased payments) received minus the tax, donation, or transfer paid to Medicaid.

Although it seems likely that most hospitals gained from DSH programs, for a variety of reasons it is more difficult to ascertain the overall impact of these programs on hospital status. First, since many of the affected hospitals (or mental facilities) were publicly owned and subsidized, the net gain to the hospital may be offset by a reduction in other budget support. As the intergovernmental and intragovernmental transfers become more dominant in special financing schemes, this is an important consideration. Second, in some cases DSH programs were established as settlements to Boren Amendment lawsuits that might have otherwise forced Medicaid to increase hospital payments. Thus, some hospitals may have had increased payments anyway, even with no DSH program. Third, if the special financing programs were not available, states might have been forced to cut Medicaid spending, which could have affected hospitals in other ways.

Similarly, in principle, a state's (in contrast to single provider's) *direct gain* from these programs is the difference of special revenues received minus the state share of DSH payments (and of other payment increases). Again, the overall impact is difficult to discern. First, this does not include state savings among state-owned hospitals or facilities that appear outside the Medicaid budget. In many states it is possible that this savings outweighs the direct gain within Medicaid. Second, some of the money saved by states was used to support other Medicaid spending growth. If these additional revenues had not been available, it is difficult to say what states would have done. Some states would still have expanded their programs owing to federal mandates and would have had to cut spending in other sectors or raise taxes. Other states might have slashed Medicaid spending.

Finally, although DSH programs increased payments to hospitals, the extent to which this resulted in more or better care for low-income patients is unclear. There are some anecdotal instances in which DSH funds were used to pay for clinics or other health care initiatives. However, if the extra funds received by a hospital simply reduced its debt, then there might not be a perceptible increase in health care delivery. Alternatively, a hospital receiving DSH money might reduce its charges to private payers, essentially transferring the savings to private payers.

SUMMARY

Throughout the past decade, Medicaid expenditures grew faster than state revenues, so that Medicaid consumed an ever larger portion of state budgets. Starting in the late 1980s, as Medicaid spending soared and state revenues flattened during the recent recession, the situation became even more problematic for states. A critical strategy employed by most states attempted to leverage more federal Medicaid dollars. The two principal leveraging strategies were "Medicaid maximization"—shifting state-only programs into Medicaid—and special financing programs, including provider tax, donation, intergovernmental transfer, and DSH programs. Even so, after netting out special revenues, it appeared that average state expenditures for Medicaid rose 17 percent per year from 1990 to 1992, still a rapid growth rate. This growth rate occurred *despite* the fact that most states undertook serious cost-containment programs in the late 1980s and early 1990s. As Medicaid grew, other parts of the state budget tended to shrink, especially higher education and discretionary programs. Many states also raised taxes, including general taxes and "sin" taxes to pay for Medicaid.

The Medicaid Voluntary Donations and Provider-Specific Tax Amendments of 1991 essentially cap these special financing programs beginning in 1993. Even though states often had difficulty enacting broad-based health care taxes, they have often been able to use inter- or intragovernmental transfers to maintain their DSH programs. Preliminary 1993 data suggest that Medicaid growth has been more than halved from the 1992 level, largely due to the DSH caps (Health Care Financing Administration, Office of the Actuary, personal communication, 1994). However, states will still have to cope with real cost increases due to continuing health care cost inflation, the aging of the population, and continuing implementation of Medicaid expansions for children and QMBs. For the short term, states will continue to face hard choices in how to contain Medicaid costs and how to cut other sectors of the budget.

The use of special financing programs and Medicaid maximization show the ingenuity of state administrators in coping with tough fiscal times. However, while these policies helped solve their budgetary problems, it is important to realize that the allocation of billions of dollars was driven by accounting procedures that shifted costs to the federal government, rather than by public policy or medical decision-making processes about how to shape better or more efficient health care systems. While states responded rationally to financial incentives built into Medicaid, the incentives did not necessarily lead to building a better system of health care for low income people.

In addition to the budgetary costs of the special financing programs, there were political costs, especially in federal-state relations. The federal government, particularly the HCFA and the Office of Management and Budget, opposed these programs and sought to have them outlawed as early as 1988. States argued back that the federal government had no authority to dictate how states collected revenues. Further, they noted that federal mandates had increased Medicaid costs and that they needed to find ways to pay for them. Protracted negotiations between the Bush administration, Congress, and the states (coordinated by the National Governors Association) led to the eventual passage of the 1991 legislation. The policy debate has continued to evolve. Under pressure from states, the Clinton administration agreed to ease the DSH caps that had been initially imposed by the Bush administration. Although these programs enabled states to ease some budgetary problems, intergovernmental relations were severely strained and Medicaid's reputation grew a little more tarnished. DSH payments are still viewed with suspicion and have been targeted as a principal area of Medicaid savings to help pay for the Clinton administration's national health care reform proposal.

Notes

1. State revenue data are from the series *State Government Finances* by the U.S. Bureau of the Census.

2. Data from the National Association of State Budget Officers for state fiscal year 1992 are estimates, whereas data for prior years are actual.

3. The terminology is not necessarily mutually exclusive. For example, a donation or tax program exclusively among public hospitals could also be considered an intergovernmental transfer program.

4. The usual taxonomy of these programs does not distinguish between inter- and intragovernmental transfers. We have separated them to better clarify whether the source of funds is state or local.

5. The interpretation of the legislation is based on the final regulations issued by the Health Care Financing Administration on August 13, 1993.

6. We did not net out other "intragovernmental" revenues, since these were basically still state funds. Transferring other state funds to Medicaid is equivalent in nature to the Medicaid maximization strategy discussed previously. However, there are probably some state funds counted among tax, donation, or intergovernmental transfer programs.

Chapter Six

LONG-TERM CARE SERVICES

Long-term care refers to a variety of services needed by persons who have lost some capacity for self-care because of a chronic illness or condition. The long-term care population includes people of all ages with a wide range of diagnoses and medical conditions including mental retardation, mental illness, strokes, and dementia. Long-term care consists of help with the basic activities of daily living such as bathing, dressing, meal preparation, and housekeeping. Furthermore, it can be provided in a variety of settings: the home, the community, or an institution.

Medicaid finances an array of long-term care services, both institutional and community-based. As for institutional care, the program covers care provided in nursing homes for the elderly and disabled, intermediate care in facilities for the mentally retarded (ICFs/MR), and inpatient care for the mentally ill. Community-based care services covered by Medicaid include home health and personal care.

Since its inception, Medicaid has been the largest payer of long-term care services among third-party payers. In 1992, the nation spent $76.6 billion on long-term care (nursing home and home health care). Medicaid paid for about 49 percent of the bill, whereas Medicare paid 7 percent and private insurance 1.8 percent (Burner, Waldo, and McKusick 1992). The balance was paid by individuals in direct out-of-pocket payments and other funding sources.

Since the late 1970s, long-term care was a dominant component in Medicaid, accounting for roughly half of total program expenditures. However, as discussed in chapter 2, the share of Medicaid funds spent on long-term care has declined over the last few years, largely because of the exceptionally high growth in hospital expenditures. By 1992, less than 40 percent of total program expenditures went toward paying for long-term care.

The bulk of Medicaid money spent on long-term care covers institutional services (table 6.1). In 1992, for example, nearly 87 percent,

Table 6.1 MEDICAID LONG-TERM CARE EXPENDITURES BY TYPE OF SERVICE AND ELIGIBILITY GROUP: 1984-92

Eligibility Group	Expenditures ($ 1992)				Expenditures Per Enrollee ($ 1992)				Share of Total Expenditures in 1992 (%)
	Level		Average Annual Change (%)		Level		Average Annual Change (%)		
	1984 (millions)	1992 (millions)	1984-90	1990-92	1984	1992	1984-90	1990-92	
Total									
All enrollees	23,962	43,628	6.0	13.2	956.92	1,236.21	3.8	1.6	100.0
Adult enrollees	48	158	11.9	29.1	8.22	19.18	15.2	16.3	0.4
Child enrollees	475	1,904	9.5	52.4	37.43	103.16	18.4	34.5	4.4
Aged enrollees	14,331	25,694	5.5	14.2	4,370.40	6,831.22	7.7	8.5	58.9
Blind and disabled enrollees	9,108	15,872	6.7	8.6	2,875.89	3,288.80	2.3	-1.3	36.4
Institutional									
All enrollees	22,807	37,862	4.5	12.8	910.78	1,072.82	2.8	1.3	86.8
Adult enrollees	25	92	12.6	33.9	4.26	11.16	17.4	20.6	0.2
Child enrollees	452	1,736	8.2	54.8	35.61	94.09	17.6	36.5	4.0
Aged enrollees	13,668	23,039	4.2	14.7	4,168.20	6,125.34	6.6	9.0	52.8
Blind and disabled enrollees	8,662	12,994	4.8	6.4	2,735.06	2,692.50	-0.3	-3.3	29.8
Home and Community-Based Care									
All enrollees	1,155	5,766	24.6	15.5	46.14	163.39	23.5	3.7	13.2
Adult enrollees	23	66	11.0	23.1	3.95	8.02	12.5	10.9	0.2
Child enrollees	23	167	26.4	33.1	1.82	9.07	30.7	17.5	0.4
Aged enrollees	663	2,655	22.1	9.8	202.20	705.88	23.2	4.3	6.1
Blind and disabled enrollees	446	2,878	28.2	20.5	140.83	596.30	27.2	9.5	6.6

Note: Arizona and U.S. territories are not included.

about $38 billion, of Medicaid spending for long-term care funded institutional services (in particular, nursing home care), whereas only about 13 percent of spending funded community-based services— home health, personal care, and waiver programs.

Throughout most of the 1980s, Medicaid spending for institutional care grew slowly—4.5 percent per year in real dollars. Then, beginning in 1990, spending began to rapidly accelerate, increasing nearly 13 percent each year between 1990 and 1992. Expenditure growth of community-based long-term care, by contrast, has been consistently high since 1984, but from a low base. Growth was exceptionally high during the 1980s: between 1984 and 1990, real community-based long-term care funding increased by about 25 percent each year. Although the overall rate of increase of community-based long-term care declined in 1991 and 1992, it remained high, growing an average of nearly 16 percent per year in each of those years. All eligibility groups experienced rapid expenditure growth, particularly children and the blind and disabled. Although increases have been dramatic, 1992 spending for community-based care still accounted for only 10 percent of long-term care spending.

The largest share of Medicaid long-term care funds is spent on care for the elderly, with most of the remainder going to the disabled, principally the mentally retarded and developmentally disabled. In 1992, 59 percent of long-term care funds was spent on the elderly, 36 percent on the disabled, 4.4 percent on children, and less than 1 percent on adults (table 6.1). This distribution has been relatively constant since 1984. The rest of this chapter discusses recent expenditure trends and policy changes for the four major Medicaid long-term services: nursing home care, ICFs/MR, inpatient mental health, and community-based care.

NURSING HOME CARE

Under the Medicaid program, states are required to pay for nursing home care for adults 21 years of age and older. Persons can obtain nursing home care if they need medical or nursing care, rehabilitation services, or if a disability requires institutional care. Previously, a distinction was made between types of facilities (skilled versus intermediate) in which nursing home services were provided. In 1990, however, this categorical distinction was eliminated, resulting in the more general term, nursing facilities (NFs).

As shown in table 6.2, Medicaid spent $24.3 billion on nursing home care in 1992. The bulk of these expenditures, greater than 80 percent, went to the elderly; most of the rest went to the blind and disabled. This expenditure distribution has changed little since 1984.

Rapid Expenditure Growth since 1990

After many years of modest growth in the 1980s, nursing home expenditures greatly accelerated in the early 1990s. Between 1984 and 1990, real expenditures increased an average of 4.2 percent each year (table 6.2). After 1990, Medicaid nursing home spending began to grow sharply, increasing 10.4 percent in 1991 and 12.9 percent in 1992. While expenditures increased rapidly, the number of nursing home recipients grew much more slowly: between 1990 and 1992, the number of people receiving nursing home care grew from 1.45 million to 1.57 million, an annual growth rate of 4.1 percent (Congressional Research Service 1993). This suggests that the recent spending surge in NF services has been fueled largely by increases in spending per recipient, rather than increases in the number of recipients.

Growth in spending per recipient can be attributed in part to the 1987 Omnibus Budget Reconciliation Act (OBRA) nursing home reforms. Under this law, states were required to ensure that certain quality standards—such as nurse staffing, aide training, and patient assessment—were being met. The costs associated with conforming to these standards also contributed to spending increases. In fact, as part of the reform, states had to demonstrate the costs of complying with the law; as of 1990, the Health Care Financing Administration (HCFA) had approved NF add-ons as high as $4.34 per day for compliance with the reform mandates.

Another factor contributing to the recent surge in nursing home care expenditures is the increasing role the courts are playing in determining Medicaid service payment rates. As described earlier, the Boren Amendment mandates that Medicaid reimbursement rates be reasonable and adequate for efficiently and economically operated facilities. A number of providers have brought lawsuits challenging that states are not meeting these mandates. According to the American Health Care Association, as of June 1992, 13 Boren Amendment suits involving nursing homes had been resolved and another 8 were pending. For most of the decided cases, the courts have instructed states to revise their payment schedules to comply with the amendment. Although it is clear that Boren suits have affected Medicaid payment rates, it is difficult to precisely measure the overall impact

Table 6.2 MEDICAID NURSING FACILITY EXPENDITURES BY ELIGIBILITY GROUP AND CASH ASSISTANCE STATUS: 1984–92

Eligibility Group	Expenditures ($ 1992)				Expenditures per Recipient[a] ($ 1992)				Share of Expenditures in 1992 (%)
	Level		Average Annual Change (%)		Level		Average Annual Change (%)		
	1984 (millions)	1992 (millions)	1984–90	1990–92	1984	1992	1984–90	1990–92	
Total	15,253	24,313	4.2	11.7	11,253	15,593	2.9	8.1	100.0
Cash assistance	2,965	3,635	1.0	7.4	11,203	17,087	4.3	8.9	14.9
Non-cash assistance	12,288	20,678	4.9	12.5	11,265	15,357	2.6	8.1	85.1
Aged	12,427	20,239	4.4	12.3	10,680	15,248	3.3	8.3	83.2
Cash assistance	1,700	1,904	−0.2	6.6	10,215	15,729	3.7	11.3	7.8
Non-cash assistance	10,728	18,335	5.0	12.9	10,757	15,200	3.3	8.0	75.4
Blind and Disabled	2,796	4,002	3.3	8.6	12,146	18,292	4.4	8.0	16.5
Cash assistance	1,259	1,713	2.5	8.2	12,804	19,496	4.9	6.8	7.0
Non-cash assistance	1,537	2,289	3.9	8.9	11,655	17,484	4.0	8.8	9.4
Other	31	72	8.7	19.3	6,266	9,823	8.7	−2.6	0.3
Cash assistance	6	17	10.1	22.3	4,931	4,551	16.5	−39.3	0.1
Non-cash assistance	24	54	8.3	18.3	6,754	15,483	6.5	25.2	0.2

Note: Arizona and U.S. territories are not included.
a. Expenditures per recipient are only for enrollees who actually received SNF (Skilled Nursing Facility) services.

they have had on nursing home expenditures. Indeed, even states that have not actually been sued have felt that the mere threat of litigation has markedly affected how and at what level they pay providers (Holahan et al. 1992).

Provider tax and donation programs could also explain part of the recent acceleration in nursing home spending. Although hospitals were by far the major provider group that participated in special revenue programs, a few states taxed nursing homes and subsequently boosted payment rates. Like the nursing home reforms and the Boren Amendment, though, it is difficult to fully evaluate the fiscal impact of special revenue programs.

Finally, the practice of Medicaid estate planning might have contributed to the recent NF expenditure surge as well. This is discussed in the following subsection.

Most Nursing Facility Funds Are Spent on the Non–cash-Assisted Elderly

Whereas more than four-fifths of Medicaid nursing facility funds are spent on the elderly, three-quarters of those funds are spent on the non–cash-assisted elderly (principally comprising the medically needy and the categorically needy with no cash assistance).[1] The share of funds spent on the non–cash-assisted elderly has been steadily rising: in 1984, spending on this population elderly accounted for 70 percent of nursing home funds; by 1992, this proportion had risen to 75 percent. In addition, the expenditure growth of the non–cash-assisted elderly has consistently outpaced that of the cash-assisted, and particularly during 1990–92.

This expenditure increase can be partly explained by the rising number of non–cash-assisted elderly receiving Medicaid nursing home services. Between 1984 and 1992, for example, the number of non–cash-assisted elderly increased about 2 percent per year. By contrast, the number of cash-assisted elderly nursing home patients declined by 4 percent per year during the same period. Spending increases for the non–cash-assisted elderly can also be attributed in part to the increasing likelihood of spend-down because of higher nursing home prices or longer stays in the nursing homes. Two other factors may be the aging of the population and the rising demand for nursing home care among the elderly population.

Beyond these, the spousal impoverishment mandates contained in the 1988 Medicare Catastrophic Cost Act (MCCA) also may have fueled expenditure increases for this group. The act included provisions allowing nursing home residents whose spouses live in the community to qualify for Medicaid nursing home coverage without impoverishing their spouses. Under these new provisions, when a state determines the amount that a married nursing home patient must contribute to his or her cost of care, a specified portion of the couple's assets and income must first be set aside. Thus, for some married individuals, Medicaid is covering a greater share of their nursing home costs than it would have otherwise.

Another possible growth factor is the alleged increase in the number of nonpoor elderly who are qualifying for Medicaid nursing home coverage by sheltering or transferring their assets. Anecdotal evidence exist suggesting that asset transfer has increased sharply in recent years (Kosterlitz 1992). Many believe that the passage and later repeal of the 1988 MCCA was a principal factor in causing the purported increase of asset transfer among the elderly; that is, after the MCCA, elderly people became more knowledgeable about exactly what Medicare did and did not cover. Although a recent survey of state Medicaid officials in six states suggests that the practice of estate planning is growing rapidly, no definitive estimate is available of how widespread the practice is at present (Burwell 1993).

INTERMEDIATE CARE FACILITIES FOR THE MENTALLY RETARDED

Since the 1970s, the Medicaid program has been a major funding source for individuals with mental retardation and related conditions such as cerebral palsy and epilepsy. Institutional Medicaid services for the developmentally disabled are mainly provided through intermediate care facilities for the mentally retarded. About three-quarters of beneficiaries of ICFs/MR are served in large state facilities. An increasing number, however, are being cared for in smaller, community-based facilities that are state or privately operated.

During the late 1970s, spending for ICFs/MR was a principal growth factor. Between 1978 and 1984, for example, ICF/MR spending grew at an average annual rate of 23.2 percent (nominal dollars)—twice the growth of overall Medicaid spending during the period. By 1984, ICF/MR expenditures accounted for about 11 percent of total Medicaid spending. The number of recipients also grew rapidly during this time, from 107,000 in 1978 to nearly 140,000 in 1984. The principal reason for this rapid growth was the passage of legislation in 1971

Table 6.3 MEDICAID EXPENDITURES FOR INTERMEDIATE CARE FACILITIES
FOR THE MENTALLY RETARDED, BY ELIGIBILITY GROUP: 1984–92

| | Expenditures ($ 1992) | | | | |
| | Level | | Average Annual Change (%) | | Share of Expenditures in 1992 (%) |
Eligibility Group	1984 (millions)	1992 (millions)	1984– 90	1990– 92	
All enrollees	5,903	8,696	5.8	2.6	100.0
Adult enrollees	1	14	40.6	26.7	0.2
Child enrollees	94	44	−0.6	−30.4	0.5
Aged enrollees	134	526	20.9	12.1	6.0
Blind and disabled enrollees	5,674	8,112	5.3	2.3	93.3

Note: Arizona and U.S. territories are not included.

authorizing Medicaid funding for care provided in ICFs/MR. Previously, states had been the principal payers of care in ICFs/MR. States quickly adopted this optional service. By 1977, just six years after the enabling legislation was passed, 43 states had elected to cover ICF/MR care.

In recent years, expenditure growth for ICFs/MR has been much slower (table 6.3). Between 1984 and 1990, spending for ICFs/MR grew at an annual rate of 5.8 percent in real dollars, or 10 percent in nominal dollars. From 1990 to 1992, expenditure increases were slower still—2.6 percent per year in real dollars. In addition, payments to ICFs/MR represent a decreasing share of overall Medicaid spending. In 1992, spending for ICFs/MR was $8.7 billion, about 7.7 percent of total Medicaid spending, down from 12 percent in 1984. Although expenditure growth has slowed, the growth in the number of persons receiving ICF/MR services has been slower still: between 1984 and 1992 recipient growth averaged less than 1 percent per year (Congressional Research Service, 1993). As a result, spending per recipient has been rising.

Several factors have contributed to this increase in expenditures per recipient. The continuing movement to deinstitutionalize the mentally retarded has caused the number of people in large state ICF/MR institutions to sharply decrease (Lakin and Hall 1990a). However, the fixed costs of running such institutions have continued to rise, and these costs are distributed across fewer and fewer patients, causing costs per patient to increase. Facility upgrading (improving staff ratios, physical plant, and the like), which was required to meet new certification standards, also contributed to expenditure growth.

Finally, as states have moved people into noninstitutional settings, patients remaining in ICFs/MR, particularly large ones, are the more profoundly disabled and thus require more costly care.

Whereas most states provide ICF/MR coverage, the states differ considerably in terms of how heavily they use the ICF/MR program. A 1988 survey of 10 states, for example, revealed that some states care for most of their developmental disabled populations in ICFs/MR, whereas others use the service sparingly. In Texas, 92 percent of the developmental disabled population used ICFs/MR, whereas Connecticut cared for only 28 percent of its developmental disabled in ICFs/MR (Lakin et al. 1989; Lakin et al. 1990b).

There is also considerable variation among the states as to the size of facilities in which they serve their developmentally disabled population. In 1988, nearly half of ICF/MR beneficiaries received care in small (less than 15 patients) community-based facilities (Lakin and Hall, 1990). This fraction, however, varied greatly from state to state. New Hampshire, for example, cared for nearly 90 percent of its ICF/MR residents in 1988 in small facilities. At the other extreme, in Mississippi only 14 percent of the developmentally disabled population was cared for in small facilities. Nationally, however, the trend is to increasingly provide ICF/MR care in small, community facilities as opposed to large state institutions (Lakin and Hall, 1990).

INSTITUTIONAL MENTAL HEALTH SERVICES

Medicaid covers two types of inpatient mental health institutions— institutions for mental disease and inpatient psychiatric hospitals. Coverage is extended to persons under age 21 or over 65; persons between ages 21 and 65 are not covered, even if they are categorically eligible for Medicaid. Why adults are excluded from inpatient mental health care is not entirely clear. Some observers have speculated that when Congress established the mental health benefit they wanted the states to continue to have some financial responsibility for caring for the mentally ill. (Prior to inpatient mental health care being offered as a Medicaid benefit, states financed such care using largely their own funds.)

One consequence of the age restriction imposed by the mental health benefit is that many adult mentally ill persons were being cared for by Medicaid under the general NF benefit. Estimates from the 1985 National Nursing Home Survey indicated that nearly

150,000 Medicaid institutionalized recipients had a primary diagnosis of mental illness, yet program data in that year show that only 77,000 persons received Medicaid inpatient mental health care in that year.

Concern about mentally ill persons being inappropriately placed in regular nursing home facilities, in addition to the concern that Medicaid was inadvertently paying for inpatient mental health care for adults, prompted Congress to include provisions in the OBRA 87 nursing home reform law requiring states to implement preadmission screening and evaluation programs for the mentally ill in nursing homes to verify they were appropriately placed.[2]

Rapid Expenditure Growth since 1990

After an extended period of modest growth—3 percent each year—in the mid-1980s, inpatient mental health spending rapidly accelerated over the years 1990–92 (table 6.4). Expenditures grew nearly 20 percent in 1991, and in 1992 they grew a record 105 percent, reaching $4.9 billion. The number of beneficiaries, by contrast, remained relatively constant throughout the 1980s.

Most of this recent expenditure surge can be attributed to states' introduction of disproportionate-share (DSH) programs for inpatient mental health services. Modeled directly after hospital DSH programs, a number of states have applied to amend their state plans to allow for collection of mental health DSH payments. Beginning in 1991, several states submitted requests to the HCFA to revise their state plans so that DSH payments made for Medicaid recipients being treated in psychiatric facilities could receive federal matching. Among the first states to establish mental health DSH programs were New Hampshire, Kansas, and Indiana. As shown in table 6.5, many other states quickly followed.

HOME AND COMMUNITY-BASED CARE

In 1992, Medicaid spent $5.8 billion on home and community-based long-term care programs: $2.3 billion on personal care, $1.3 billion on home health, and $2.2 billion on home and community-based waiver programs (table 6.6). Through the 1980s, Medicaid expenditures for community-based care increased dramatically: between

Table 6.4 MEDICAID MENTAL HEALTH EXPENDITURES BY ELIGIBILITY GROUP: 1984–92

Eligibility Group	Expenditures ($ 1992) Level		Average Annual Change (%)		Expenditures per Recipient[a] ($ 1992) Level		Average Annual Change (%)		Share of Expenditures in 1992 (%)
	1984 (millions)	1992 (millions)	1984–90	1990–92	1984	1992	1984–90	1990–92	
All recipients	1,650	4,853	3.2	56.2	46,642	63,328	−12.1	71.4	100.0
Adult recipients	13	30	4.3	35.5	5,909	15,453	−12.2	138.6	0.6
Child recipients	339	1,668	10.3	65.4	25,337	42,208	−6.0	55.3	34.4
Aged recipients	1,106	2,275	−1.1	48.0	74,881	116,017	−7.2	55.7	46.9
Blind and disabled recipients	192	880	9.2	64.4	29,346	57,854	−15.1	129.2	18.1

Note: Arizona and U.S. territories are not included.

a. Expenditures per recipient are only for enrollees who actually received mental health services.

Table 6.5 INPATIENT MENTAL HEALTH EXPENDITURES AND GROWTH RATES, BY STATES: 1984-92

	Expenditures ($ 1992, thousands)				Average Annual Growth Rate (%)		
	1984	1990	1991	1992	1984-90	1990-91	1991-92
Alabama	1,452	6,637	13,247	21,091	28.7	99.4	59.8
Alaska	1,887	856	775	795	-12.5	-9.6	3.0
Arkansas	63	17,998	16,436	26,859	156.3	-8.8	64.0
California	0	1,652	245	1,418	0.0	-85.2	480.2
Colorado	14,630	14,953	19,599	20,908	0.2	30.9	7.1
Connecticut	33,185	36,293	43,003	165,547	1.4	18.4	286.4
Delaware	2,416	1,947	0	0	-3.7	0.0	0.0
District of Columbia	31,009	30,813	29,296	41,541	-0.2	-5.0	42.3
Florida	8,937	10,883	12,261	13,372	3.2	12.6	9.5
Georgia	0	0	0	0	0.0	0.0	0.0
Hawaii	0	0	0	0	0.0	0.0	0.0
Idaho	0	625	2,613	951	0.0	317.8	-63.5
Illinois	21,193	19,564	21,587	26,025	-1.4	10.2	21.0
Indiana	3,078	23,998	53,539	91,639	40.6	122.9	71.8
Iowa	2,885	11,641	12,282	17,166	26.0	5.4	40.3
Kansas	15,439	22,588	80,165	208,127	6.4	254.5	160.6
Kentucky	13,824	44,581	27,023	34,210	21.4	-39.4	27.1
Louisiana	10,689	50,411	51,868	49,188	29.3	2.8	-4.8
Maine	0	6,144	7,393	46,092	0.0	20.2	525.7
Maryland	32,497	12,074	9,829	56,222	-15.3	-18.7	474.1
Massachusetts	6,321	3,230	22,515	34,990	-10.7	596.4	56.0
Michigan	65,869	155,230	142,232	161,538	15.2	-8.5	14.0
Minnesota	15,291	36,716	37,618	36,981	15.6	2.4	-1.3
Mississippi	0	0	0	9,763	0.0	0.0	0.0

Missouri	20,351	8,314	10,848	259,038	−14.0	30.4	2296.5
Montana	0	10,058	10,907	13,714	0.0	8.3	26.2
Nebraska	4,957	5,871	6,632	8,391	2.7	12.9	27.0
Nevada	274	273	637	5,607	−0.2	133.3	783.8
New Hampshire	4,998	6,874	28,572	44,084	5.3	315.2	54.9
New Jersey	82,418	50,105	141,202	693,432	−8.1	181.5	392.9
New Mexico	0	0	234	14,258	0.0	0.0	6028.1
New York	826,921	833,177	891,329	1,255,884	0.0	6.9	41.4
North Carolina	15,187	38,944	44,186	45,808	16.8	13.4	4.1
North Dakota	5,870	3,232	3,679	1,677	−9.6	13.7	−54.3
Ohio	67,943	66,722	107,136	127,382	−0.4	60.4	19.3
Oklahoma	10,881	44,516	47,588	75,069	26.3	6.8	58.3
Oregon	8,421	11,807	13,769	16,136	5.7	16.5	17.6
Pennsylvania	218,347	234,054	236,686	883,074	1.0	1.0	274.5
Rhode Island	2,315	7,667	8,031	11,910	21.9	4.6	48.9
South Carolina	14,322	29,973	43,098	68,461	13.0	43.6	59.4
South Dakota	3,807	4,275	4,640	5,404	1.8	8.4	16.9
Tennessee	22,137	37,773	30,484	33,429	9.2	−19.4	10.1
Texas	0	0	0	0	0.0	0.0	0.0
Utah	7,195	6,453	6,043	6,667	−1.9	−6.4	10.7
Vermont	1,108	534	564	10,550	−11.5	5.4	1778.5
Virginia	22,735	29,327	50,033	70,236	4.2	70.4	40.9
Washington	4,796	17,102	31,623	92,894	23.5	84.7	194.8
West Virginia	0	3,928	6,817	9,970	0.0	73.4	46.8
Wisconsin	24,388	29,482	34,446	34,904	3.1	16.7	1.7
Wyoming	0	415	548	698	0.0	32.0	28.0
U.S. total	1,650,039	1,989,708	2,363,258	4,853,096	3.0	18.7	106.1

Note: Arizona and U.S. territories are not included.

Table 6.6 MEDICAID HOME AND COMMUNITY-BASED CARE EXPENDITURES, BY TYPE OF SERVICE: 1984–92

| Type of Service | Expenditures ($ 1992) | | | | Expenditures per Enrollee ($ 1992) | | | | Share of Expenditures in 1992 (%) |
| | Level | | Average Annual Change (%) | | Level | | Average Annual Change (%) | | |
	1984 (millions)	1992 (millions)	1984–90	1990–92	1984	1992	1984–90	1990–92	
Total home health	1,155	5,766	24.6	15.5	46.14	161.73	22.0	3.1	100.0
Personal care	0	2,340	—	6.8	0.00	65.61	—	–4.7	40.6
HCB[a] waivers	458	2,153	20.1	25.1	18.29	60.38	17.6	11.6	37.3
Home health	697	1,254	4.3	18.2	27.85	35.16	2.1	5.5	21.7
Other	0	21	—[b]	—	0.00	0.58	—	—	0.4

Notes: Arizona and U.S. territories are not included. Dashes (—) denote rates that cannot be computed due to division by zero.
a. HCB, home and community-based.
b. Not applicable.

Table 6.7 MEDICAID EXPENDITURES FOR HOME AND COMMUNITY-BASED
CARE, BY ELIGIBILITY GROUP: 1984–92

| | Expenditures ($ 1992) | | | | |
| | Level | | Average Annual Change (%) | | Share of Expenditures in 1992 (%) |
Eligibility Group	1984 (millions)	1992 (millions)	1984– 90	1990– 92	
All enrollees	1,155	5,766	24.6	15.5	100.0
Adult enrollees	23	91	18.1	19.9	1.6
Child enrollees	23	209	32.4	29.5	3.6
Aged enrollees	663	2,468	21.0	9.0	42.8
Blind and disabled enrollees	446	2,999	29.0	20.8	52.0

Note: Arizona and U.S. territories are not included.

1984 and 1990, real spending grew at an annual rate of 24.6 percent.
Although increases have slowed in the 1990s, expenditure growth
still remains high, averaging 15.5 percent per year.

This rapid growth partly reflects the continued general movement
toward noninstitutional services for the long-term care population.
That is, beginning in the late 1970s there was a widespread consensus
among practitioners, patient advocates, and policymakers that long-
term care (for certain segments of the long-term care population)
could be better provided in the community as opposed to an institution. It also reflects the development of home and community-based
waiver programs that were adopted by states throughout the 1980s.
The bulk of the expenditure growth occurred in the two optional
programs—the personal care program and the waiver program.
Whereas home health spending increased, the rate was far below
that for personal care or the waiver programs.

Mirroring the rapid expenditure growth, the number of beneficiaries receiving community-based care swelled from 437,000 in 1984
to 926,000 in 1992. Most of the funds spent on community-based
care went toward care for the blind and disabled; the remainder went
toward care for the elderly (table 6.7). In 1992, the blind and disabled
represented 52 percent of community-based spending, the elderly
43 percent, and adults and children combined only about 5 percent.

Medicaid's main community-based programs—personal care,
home health, and waiver programs—differ in design and focus.[3]
Home health is a mandatory Medicaid benefit that all states must
provide to persons over age 21. Provided only through agencies, the

home health benefit has a strong medical orientation and is structured much like Medicare's home health benefit.

Despite being the first community-based program offered by Medicaid, home health is the smallest of the three main community-based programs. Some attribute this to the states' reluctance to use the full home health benefit (Feder 1988). As mentioned previously, this benefit provides principally skilled home care services. Unlike Medicare, though, the Medicaid home health benefit does not require states to make eligibility for home health care contingent upon the person being homebound. States, however, are given considerable latitude in the actual design of the benefit. Because states are fearful of the cost implications of a broad home care program, they have adopted various methods to limit the home health benefit, including restricting visits, limiting services to skilled care, and limiting provider payments. This has effectively enabled the states to both restrict the amount of home health care provided as well as limit the type of care provided to skilled care. The bulk of Medicaid spending for home health goes to provide services to the elderly.

Personal care, the largest of Medicaid's three community-based programs, is an optional service under Medicaid. Typically, it consists of help with personal care such as bathing, dressing, and eating as well as help with housekeeping duties such as meal preparation and shopping. In contrast with home health, personal care can be provided by individuals as well as agencies. In 1992, 28 states covered personal care. Personal care, for any person who was entitled to Medicaid nursing home care, was scheduled to become a mandatory benefit under Medicaid in 1994, but this mandate was repealed in the OBRA 93.

States can also offer community-based long-term care services through various waiver authorities.[4] In a nutshell, states can apply to the federal government for authorization to provide home and community-based care. Most often, waiver programs are targeted to persons who would otherwise receive Medicaid care in an institution. Prompted by concern that Medicaid had too strong of an institutional bias, the first of the community-based waivers was established in the Omnibus Budget Reconciliation Act 1981 and was termed the Medicaid Home and Community-Based Services Program. Less formally, it has become known as the "2176 waiver program" (after the section in OBRA 81) or the "1915(c) waiver program" (after the section of the Social Security Act). Through this waiver, states are allowed to provide a wide range of home and community-based care services (including homemaker, personal care, and case management) to the elderly, the mentally retarded, and other chronically ill populations. Although the 1915(c) waiver was initially targeted to persons at risk of being institutionalized, it has since been amended so that persons with other chronic conditions—such as AIDS—can be covered. Services provided in 1915(c) waiver programs must be budget neutral; that is, the state must demonstrate that the average cost per waiver participant does not exceed what Medicaid would have spent on participants had the waiver program not been implemented.

The other major community-based care waiver program was established by OBRA 87 and is referred to as the "1915(d) waiver program." Unlike the 1915(c) program, the 1915(d) program is targeted expressly to elderly persons age 65 and over who are at risk of being institutionalized. The budget neutrality requirement was eliminated in the 1915(d) program; instead, a cap was placed on the state's total Medicaid long-term care expenditures. At present, Oregon is the only state that has implemented a 1915(d) waiver program.

Waiver programs (like the 1915(c) and 1915(d) programs) offer states numerous advantages over both the home health benefit and the personal care option. Perhaps the most important advantage is that waiver programs greatly limit states' risk. Under waiver programs, states can offer services to a specific geographic area and to select groups of Medicaid eligibles, for example, those that would otherwise require institutional care. By contrast, both the home health benefit and personal care option require that the service be provided to all eligible persons in the state. Some believe that this open-ended entitlement feature greatly hampered the development of the home health and personal care programs. The waiver programs also allow states to apply the more generous institutional eligibility financial standards (such as the "300 percent rule" described previously—see note 1), rather than the usual Medicaid income standards applied to persons living in the community.

Almost all states offer community-based care through the 1915(c) waiver option. In 1991, states operated a total of 167 waiver programs that served more than 185,000 persons. In that year, nearly three-quarters of these persons were aged and disabled; most of the rest, about one-fifth, were mentally retarded or developmentally disabled. While the aged and disabled represented an overwhelming share of participants, they accounted for only 31 percent of program spending. The mentally retarded/developmentally disabled, by contrast, accounted for 65 percent of spending (Miller 1992). This seeming anomaly can be explained by the exceptionally high costs of caring for the developmentally disabled in waiver programs. Only a small fraction of waiver funds goes to serve other populations such as disabled children, persons with AIDS, and the mentally ill.

There is considerable variation in the extent to which states provide community-based care (table 6.8). In 1992, for example, community-based care accounted for over 30 percent of Oregon's total long-term care spending. New York also spent a large share of its long-term care budget on such care. (New York also spends by far the most on community-based care; in 1992, it paid $2.3 billion on community-based services, nearly 40 percent of the national Medicaid spending for such services.) By contrast, other states such as California, Louisiana, and Mississippi spend very little of their Medicaid long-term care budgets on community-based care.

States also vary as to the types of community-based care programs they provide. In 1992, Arkansas, Idaho, Michigan, New York, and Texas, for example, spent 50 percent or more of their community-based funds on personal care. Other states, by contrast, spent the bulk of their community-based funds on waiver programs. In fact, seven states (Illinois, New Hampshire, North Dakota, Oregon, Rhode Island, Utah, and Wyoming) spent more than 90 percent of their funds on waiver services.

SUMMARY

Since the early 1980s, several important shifts have occurred in Medicaid spending for and use of long-term care services. Most prominently, community-based long-term care expenditures rapidly grew: between 1984 and 1990, spending for such care increased by some 25 percent each year, after accounting for inflation. Although the rate of spending growth has declined since 1990, it still remains high, at about 16 percent a year. Much of this increase can be attributed to the growth in the personal care and waiver programs. Despite this exceptionally fast expenditure rise, community-based care represents only 10 percent of total Medicaid long-term care spending, about what it represented in 1984.

States vary widely in the degree to which they provide community-based long-term care: some states place considerable emphasis on community-based care and spend a large portion of their total long-term care budget on such care. By contrast, several states continue to rely almost exclusively on institutional long-term care services.

Table 6.8 COMMUNITY-BASED LONG-TERM CARE EXPENDITURES, BY STATE AND TYPE OF EXPENDITURE: 1992

	1992 Community-Based Expenditures as Percentage of Total LTC[a] Expenditures	Total 1992 Expenditures for Community-Based LTC Services ($ Thousands)	Percentage of Total		
			Home and Community-Based Waivers	Home Health Care	Personal Care
Alabama	11.4	53,187	73.2	26.8	0.0
Alaska	3.4	1,764	0.0	30.2	69.8
Arkansas	13.6	54,921	11.6	11.2	77.2
California	2.4	49,289	67.9	32.1	0.0
Colorado	21.1	80,062	88.7	11.3	0.0
Connecticut	14.9	183,353	71.5	28.5	0.0
Delaware	17.1	16,658	51.7	48.3	0.0
District of Columbia	5.4	13,157	0.0	59.0	41.0
Florida	8.0	94,312	45.4	53.2	1.4
Georgia	11.5	78,924	53.6	46.4	0.0
Hawaii	9.2	10,495	88.5	11.5	0.0
Idaho	12.7	14,477	37.3	7.9	54.8
Illinois	7.3	123,756	90.3	9.7	0.0
Indiana	3.5	36,650	8.1	91.9	0.0
Iowa	4.3	16,986	11.4	88.6	0.0
Kansas	6.2	31,065	75.3	14.9	9.8
Kentucky	18.0	86,445	37.9	62.1	0.0
Louisiana	2.4	18,325	14.3	85.7	0.0
Maine	10.0	37,642	67.3	24.2	8.5
Maryland	19.3	120,938	68.3	14.9	16.8
Massachusetts	14.0	258,675	42.1	27.4	30.6
Michigan	16.8	192,994	31.8	8.4	59.9
Minnesota	15.5	185,789	55.2	9.9	34.9
Mississippi	2.3	7,380	16.2	83.8	0.0
Missouri	8.5	85,375	72.2	5.4	22.4
Montana	20.9	24,943	66.9	6.1	27.0
Nebraska	15.2	36,284	66.0	25.8	8.2

(continued)

Table 6.8 COMMUNITY-BASED LONG-TERM CARE EXPENDITURES, BY STATE AND TYPE OF EXPENDITURE: 1992

	1992 Community-Based Expenditures as Percentage of Total LTC[a] Expenditures	Total 1992 Expenditures for Community-Based LTC Services ($ Thousands)	Percentage of Total		
			Home and Community-Based Waivers	Home Health Care	Personal Care
Nevada	10.8	9,982	47.1	37.0	15.9
New Hampshire	22.5	55,448	94.4	2.9	2.7
New Jersey	11.5	235,277	56.1	29.4	14.6
New Mexico	13.9	23,785	81.5	18.5	0.0
New York	24.2	2,113,255	0.8	20.6	78.7
North Carolina	13.3	124,847	40.2	36.5	23.2
North Dakota	15.2	23,010	90.3	9.7	0.0
Ohio	3.3	67,550	68.3	31.7	0.0
Oklahoma	12.5	59,291	45.9	0.4	53.8
Oregon	33.8	129,101	92.8	0.9	6.3
Pennsylvania	5.4	176,669	79.5	20.5	0.0
Rhode Island	16.3	56,081	95.5	4.5	0.0
South Carolina	7.7	36,371	80.7	18.5	0.8
South Dakota	15.7	19,839	85.6	7.3	7.1
Tennessee	7.6	46,926	69.4	30.6	0.0
Texas[b]	11.0	178,824	9.9	2.8	75.9
Utah	21.3	29,582	91.7	6.2	2.1
Vermont	23.1	26,301	86.2	13.8	0.0
Virginia	10.6	67,663	77.3	22.7	0.0
Washington	16.0	127,906	83.0	5.2	11.8
West Virginia	22.8	63,863	43.6	18.9	37.5
Wisconsin[b]	16.9	169,405	46.3	41.4	12.2
Wyoming	23.9	11,576	91.2	8.8	0.0
United States	13.2	5,766,398	37.3	21.8	40.7

Note: Arizona is not included.
a. LTC, long-term care.
b. Total includes expenditures for "other" long-term care.

States also vary as to the types of community-based services they provide. Some fund primarily personal care services, whereas others fund primarily waiver services.

Another important shift that has occurred is the recent expenditure surge for nursing home care. After an extended period of modest growth (averaging 4.2 percent between 1984 and 1990 in constant terms), Medicaid spending for nursing facilities accelerated between 1990 and 1992, growing more than 8 percent per year in constant dollars. By contrast, recipient growth over that period was only about 4 percent per year. Thus, the expenditure rise has been occasioned by increases in spending per recipient rather than increases in number of recipients. A variety of factors have contributed to the recent growth in spending per recipient, including the OBRA 87 nursing home reforms, the Boren Amendment, and special financing programs. The practice of Medicaid estate planning may also be a contributing factor.

The alleged rise in estate planning may also partly account for the growing number of non–cash-assisted elderly persons receiving Medicaid nursing home coverage: between 1984 and 1992, the number of non–cash-assisted elderly persons increased by about 2 percent each year. By contrast, the number of cash-assisted elderly nursing home recipients declined by 4 percent a year over the period. In addition to estate planning, the growth in the non–cash-assisted elderly may also reflect the aging of the overall population and the impact of the spousal impoverishment mandates, among other things.

Yet another shifting trend in Medicaid long-term care spending patterns has been the declining prominence of the ICF/MR benefit. During the later 1970s, spending for ICFs/MR was a major expenditure growth factor, increasing at twice the rate of overall Medicaid spending. In recent years, however, ICF/MR expenditure growth has been considerably slower: between 1984 and 1990, spending grew at an annual rate of 5.8 percent in constant dollars; over the 1990–92 time period, spending increases declined to less than 3 percent a year.

Notes

1. Elderly persons typically gain Medicaid NF coverage in one of three ways. They can be categorically eligible, that is they qualify for SSI and thus are entitled to NF coverage as well as cash assistance through the SSI program. Alternatively, if they live in a state with a medically needy program that covers long-term care for the elderly, they can qualify for NF care by depleting their assets and income levels to

the point that they meet needy standards set by the state. Persons who qualify by asset depletion are the so-called spend-down population. Finally, in some states elderly persons can obtain NF coverage if their income falls below 300 percent of the basic SSI benefit ($1,302 in 1993), the "300 percent rule." The medically needy and "300 percent rule" populations thus receive NF coverage but not cash assistance.

2. The OBRA 90 contained amendments to these provisions. Specifically, the OBRA 90 narrowed the definition of mental illness so that persons with a nonprimary diagnosis of dementia or a primary diagnosis that was not a serious illness did not have to be screened or evaluated as prescribed under the OBRA 87.

3. OBRA 90 established a new, optional Medicaid home care service. It is often referred to as the "frail elderly program" or "4711 provisions." Under this program, states can provide home and community services to disabled aged persons. To qualify for the program, an elderly individual must be unable to perform with human help at least two of three activities of daily living—toileting, transferring, and eating. Persons can also qualify if they are cognitively impaired. Unlike any other Medicaid benefit, federal expenditures are capped at a predetermined level each year. As of 1992, only Texas and Rhode Island had gained approval to provide care under the frail elderly program option.

4. Here we limit our discussion to two waiver authorities, 1915(c) and 1915(d). Other important waiver programs include the 1915(e) waiver, the 1915(c) model waivers, and the 1115(a) waiver.

Under the 1915(e) waiver, which was included as part of the 1988 MCCA, states are given the option to provide community care to children under the age of 5 who are infected with the AIDS virus and who would otherwise need Medicaid institutional care. The 1915(c) model waiver program, established in 1982 (one year after the regular 1915(c) waiver program), is designed to help overcome problems select disabled populations, particularly disabled children, encounter in securing eligibility for Medicaid. In essence, under 1915(c) model waiver programs, states are allowed to modify the way financial resources are counted in determining Medicaid eligibility. Beyond these specific targeted waiver programs, the Department of Health and Human Services has been granted broad authority to waive Medicaid law so that states may conduct demonstration projects that are "likely to assist in promoting the objectives" of the program. Perhaps the best known of the 1115(a) demonstration waivers is the Arizona Health Care Cost Containment System (AHCCCS).

Chapter Seven

ACUTE AND PREVENTIVE
MEDICAL SERVICES

In most states Medicaid offers a broad package of acute and preventive care benefits, providing a wider array of services than standard private insurance or Medicare. Furthermore, Medicaid does not usually require any cost sharing from its recipients—also adding to its relative generosity. However, states sometimes impose limits on amount, duration or scope of services—such as limits on hospital days or prescriptions—that delimit their generosity. States are required to offer these core services: inpatient and outpatient hospital care; physician services; laboratory and radiology; Early and Periodic Screening, Diagnostic, and Treatment services for children (EPSDT); family planning, and payment of Medicare premiums, and deductibles and copayments. States have the option of providing prescription drugs, clinic, dental, and optometry services, and numerous other services. Some optional services, such as prescription drugs, are offered by almost all states for categorically needy clients.

This chapter asks: What were the trends in expenditure patterns for Medicaid acute and preventive medical services? and What policy changes affected these services from 1984 to 1992? We specifically discuss the following services: inpatient hospital; physician, laboratory, and radiology services; outpatient hospital or clinic services; prescription drugs; EPSDT; Medicare payments; managed care; and "other" acute and preventive services. Particular emphasis is given to policy trends for inpatient hospital spending and managed care, two increasingly important topics.

As described in chapter 6, during the early 1980s Medicaid expenditure growth was dominated by long-term care. Beginning in the late 1980s this trend reversed, and spending for acute and preventive care services grew more rapidly. As shown in table 7.1, growth rates for acute and preventive care expenditures quadrupled between the 1984–90 period (6.4 percent per year in constant dollars) and the 1990–92 period (29.4 percent per year). In 1992, $64 billion was

Table 7.1 TOTAL ACUTE AND PREVENTIVE CARE: MEDICAID EXPENDITURES BY ELIGIBILITY GROUP

Eligibility Group	Expenditures ($ 1992)				Expenditures per Enrollee ($ 1992)				Share of Expenditures in 1992 (%)
	Level ($)		Average Annual Change (%)		Level ($)		Average Annual Change (%)		
	1984 (millions)	1992 (millions)	1984–90	1990–92	1984	1992	1984–90	1990–92	
All enrollees	26,478	64,375	6.4	29.4	1,057.41	1,824.07	4.2	16.2	100.0
Adult enrollees	6,721	15,314	5.8	27.5	1,139.67	1,856.52	3.6	14.8	23.8
Child enrollees	6,561	18,497	7.9	33.5	516.71	1,002.23	5.7	17.8	28.7
Aged enrollees	4,590	6,520	-0.1	19.5	1,399.75	1,733.52	-0.7	13.6	10.1
Blind and disabled enrollees	8,607	24,044	8.5	30.7	2,717.69	4,981.99	4.5	18.7	37.3

Notes: Arizona and U.S. territories are not included. Figures for all enrollees do not include payments to HMOs or to Medicare.

spent on acute and preventive care in Medicaid across the nation. The average expenditure per enrollee grew 4.2 percent per year between 1984 and 1990, and 16.2 percent per year in 1990–92.

There were two key reasons for this surge in acute and preventive care costs. First, inpatient hospital costs grew as disproportionate-share (DSH) payments ballooned. As discussed in chapter 5, the use of DSH programs for inpatient care skyrocketed during 1990–92, causing inpatient hospital costs to soar. Second, during the late 1980s the composition of the Medicaid caseload shifted: the enrollment of adults, children, and the blind and disabled grew more rapidly than that of the aged. Since the aged are dominant users of long-term care, the caseload composition shift led to a higher overall growth in acute care services. As discussed in chapter 3, the caseload shift was caused both by federal mandates and by the recent recession.

Whereas long-term care services are used primarily by the aged and disabled, acute and preventive services are critical to all types of enrollees. Even so, as seen in table 7.1 there are large differences in expenditures per enrollee. In 1992, the average expenditures per disabled enrollee ($4,982) were about three times higher than those for a non-disabled adult ($1,857) or an aged enrollee ($1,734), while children's average costs ($1,002) were about half those of an adult or aged enrollee. Adults, children, and the disabled all had similar increases in average expenditures per enrollee—consistently higher than the rate of inflation. Even though many of the new adult enrollees were pregnant women—who have relatively high medical expenses—overall the increase in expenditures per adult were similar to those for children or the disabled. However, the constant dollar expenditure per aged enrollee declined slightly in the 1984–90 period and grew less rapidly than that for other groups in the 1990–92 period. A likely explanation is that during the late 1980s, states increasingly shifted their aged Medicaid enrollees into dual enrollment in Medicaid and Medicare. Thus, during the 1980s, more of the elderly's health care costs were being paid by Medicare, so that Medicaid costs appeared to flatten.

INPATIENT HOSPITAL SERVICES

As with private health insurance and Medicare, the single largest expenditure category in Medicaid is inpatient hospital costs. As shown in table 7.2, $37.2 billion was spent in 1992, with an average cost of $1,055 per enrollee—almost double the 1984 constant dollar cost of $511 per enrollee. Even after controlling for inflation in hospital input costs, expenditure increases averaged 6.5 percent per year during 1984–90 and an incredible 41 percent per year during 1990–92. The growth of reported expenditures was especially rapid from 1990 to 1992, as DSH programs expanded. Although some of the growth was caused by rising enrollment, the main factor was increasing expenditures per enrollee. Constant dollar costs per enrollee grew 27 percent per year between 1990 and 1992.

Adults, children, and blind and disabled persons all had similar rates of growth in expenditures per enrollee, but the profile differed for the aged. Constant dollar expenditures per aged enrollee actually fell between 1984 and 1990. Although not shown, a large drop occurred in 1989, probably due to the initial implementation of the qualified medicare beneficiary (QMB) provisions. Under these provisions, Medicaid was required to cover new groups of the elderly, but only had to pay for Medicare premiums, deductibles, and copayments. Thus, enrollment of the elderly grew more quickly than the Medicaid costs. It is also plausible that some portion of the decline in average expenditures was due to actual decreases in hospital utilization among the elderly caused by Medicare's adoption of the prospective payment system for hospitals in this time period.

Reasons for Surge in Inpatient Costs

Two major policy factors contributed to the surge in inpatient costs in the late 1980s: the Boren Amendment and DSH programs. The Boren Amendment was passed in 1980 (with revisions in 1981) as an attempt to increase flexibility for nursing home and hospital payment systems, paving the way for prospective payment systems. But it also required states to demonstrate that reimbursement rates "are reasonable and adequate to meet the costs which must be incurred by efficiently and economically operated facilities."[1] During the late 1980s, hospitals and nursing homes began to file lawsuits to force state Medicaid programs to increase (or not cut) payment levels. This culminated in a 1990 Supreme Court decision in *Wilder v. Virginia Hospital Association*, which upheld hospitals' right to sue states (Wilder v. Virginia Hospital Association 1990). Based on Boren Amendment lawsuits or threats of lawsuits, many states changed reimbursement methods, increased hospital payment rates, increased

Table 7.2 HOSPITAL INPATIENT: MEDICAID EXPENDITURES BY ELIGIBILITY GROUP

	Expenditures ($ 1992)				Expenditures per Enrollee ($ 1992)				
	Level ($)		Average Annual Change (%)		Level ($)		Average Annual Change (%)		Share of Expenditures in 1992 (%)
Eligibility Group	1984 (millions)	1992 (millions)	1984–90	1990–92	1984	1992	1984–90	1990–92	
All enrollees	12,797	37,234	6.5	41.3	511.03	1,055.02	4.3	26.8	100.0
Adult enrollees	3,262	8,815	6.5	36.2	553.09	1,068.61	4.2	22.7	23.7
Child enrollees	3,081	11,069	10.1	42.0	242.66	599.78	7.9	25.3	29.7
Aged enrollees	2,004	2,959	–4.9	41.0	611.20	786.58	–5.4	34.0	7.9
Blind and disabled enrollees	4,450	14,391	7.7	44.1	1,405.02	2,981.88	3.6	30.9	38.7

Note: Arizona and U.S. territories are not included.

their inflation update factors, or developed DSH programs to boost hospital programs.

The more important reason for the recent growth in hospital expenditures is DSH programs, also discussed in chapter 5. By law, regular Medicaid payments to hospitals may not exceed Medicare levels, except those made to hospitals that provide a "disproportionate share" of care to low-income patients such as Medicaid or charity care patients. Thus, DSH policies permit enhanced payments to targeted hospitals in a state. The original intent was to recompense hospitals that might lose money due to serving a large number of Medicaid or uninsured patients. Although primarily used for acute care hospitals, DSH payments have also been used for mental health facilities by several states (Health Policy Alternatives 1992). States may have more than one DSH program, each using different rules, revenue sources, and targeted hospitals.

Until the implementation of limits of DSH under the Medicaid Voluntary Contributions and Provider-Specific Tax Amendments of 1991, states had great discretion in determining DSH hospitals and how to set DSH payment levels. As discussed in chapter 5 on financing Medicaid growth, DSH payments, in conjunction with provider taxes, donations, and intergovernmental transfers, were used to leverage greater federal contributions to Medicaid, and often artificially inflated actual Medicaid expenditures. As noted in chapter 5, the estimated level of DSH payments mushroomed from $902 million in 1990 to $17.4 billion in 1992.

Accounting for Special Revenues and DSH Payments

By incorporating data about special revenues and DSH payments, we can refine estimates of inpatient hospital expenditures to account for the net direct gains for hospitals' payments and also to reflect gains in "regular" hospital payments versus DSH payments.[2] Table 7.3 first shows the "regular reported" inpatient hospital expenditures for 1990 and 1992, then deducts special revenues (provider taxes, provider donations, and intergovernmental transfers), and then deducts the remaining DSH payments. If we assume that, in general, taxes, donations, and intergovernmental transfers made by hospitals (or on behalf of hospitals) were just "loans" that were designed to be paid back through DSH payments, then by subtracting special revenues, we can estimate the direct gains in Medicaid revenue by hospitals. Thus, an estimated $15.1 billion in DSH payments for acute inpatient care can be allocated into $7.1 billion from special

Table 7.3 HOSPITAL INPATIENT EXPENDITURES, 1990 AND 1992: EFFECT OF
EXCLUSIONS FOR SPECIAL REVENUES AND DSH PAYMENTS

Category of Expenditures	Expenditures (millions of $ 1992)	Expenditures per Enrollee ($ 1992)
1990 Inpatient Expenditures		
Regular reported expenditures	18,658	656
Excluding special revenues	18,224	641
Excluding all DSH payments	17,627	620
1992 Inpatient Expenditures		
Regular reported expenditures	37,234	1,055
Excluding special revenues	30,143	854
Excluding all DSH payments	22,104	626
Average Annual Change, 1990–92		
Regular reported expenditures	41.3%	26.8%
Excluding special revenues	28.6%	15.4%
Excluding all DSH payments	12.0%	0.5%

Note: Arizona and U.S. territories are not included.

revenue donated by providers and $8 billion in direct gain by the providers. However, as discussed in chapter 5, this does not account for other reductions in local subsidies for public hospitals or for "regular" payment increases that would have occurred in the absence of DSH programs.

Although reported data indicate that acute inpatient expenditures per enrollee rose 26.8 percent per year between 1990 and 1992 (in constant dollars), the direct gain was about half that rate—15.4 percent per year. That is, net payments to hospitals per enrollee rose 16 percent above the rate of inflation during that period. Although this was substantially less than the apparent 27 percent growth rate, it was about four times higher than the 1984–90 growth rate (see table 7.2) before the explosion in special financing programs.

We also deducted all DSH payments from inpatient hospital expenditures—reflecting the changes in "regular" hospital payments. Put this way, non-DSH inpatient expenditures per enrollee basically kept pace with inflation; the average non-DSH expenditure per enrollee grew 0.5 percent annually in constant dollars. Although DSH payments surged between 1990 and 1992, "regular" inpatient payments just kept pace with inflation.

In many cases DSH payments were negotiated between state Medicaid programs and hospitals as a substitute for regular hospital payment increases in response to Boren Amendment lawsuits or other pressures. Thus, if DSH programs did not exist at all, state Medicaid programs would probably have been forced to increase regular, non-DSH hospital payments somewhat faster than they actually did. It seems plausible that Medicaid hospital expenditures per enrollee would have climbed about 5 percent per year in constant dollars in 1990–92 if DSH programs did not exist. This estimate is derived from the facts that (1) the average historical rate of hospital expenditure growth during 1984–90 was 4.3 percent, and (2) the growth rate for physician expenditures per enrollee during 1990–92 was 5.4 percent.[3] Assuming that inpatient expenditures would have increased about 5 percent in the absence of DSH, DSH programs increased total reported Medicaid inpatient hospital costs by an additional 22 percent per year for the 1990–92 period.

Since formulae used for DSH designation or payment[4] typically include uncompensated or charity care, an important implication is that in recent years, Medicaid has been paying for large amounts of care for uninsured people. Thus, in addition to the expansions of eligibility that occurred in recent years, Medicaid was paying for hospital care for people not even on Medicaid. In 1991, it is estimated that the total level of uncompensated acute hospital care was $13 billion (CBO 1993). As noted previously, hospitals gained (in direct terms) $8.0 billion from DSH in 1992, so that DSH payments could have paid for a large share of hospitals' uncompensated care costs.

However, it is *not* clear whether the extra DSH funds led to expansions or improvements of care for uninsured or low-income people. On an anecdotal basis, some payments to DSH hospitals were used to reduce general county debt or local tax rates.[5] Other hospitals used the funds to support new clinics or services, as well as to reduce their debt burden. Even if the money is retained by hospitals and used toward uncompensated care, it is not clear that the funds would be used to provide *more* uncompensated care for uninsured people. It is also possible that reduced losses permitted DSH hospitals to reduce their charge levels to private payers (i.e., to reduce cost shifting). Thus, DSH payments could even lower prices paid by private patients.

Other Changes in Hospital Policies

The controversy about DSH programs overshadows the fact that "regular" hospital payment policies were being reformed over the past several years. States continued a long trend toward replacing retrospective payments systems with prospective payment systems such as diagnosis-related group systems or flat per diem rates. In 1985, 14 states had retrospective payment systems; this number fell to 8 by 1987 and to 4 by 1991 (Congressional Research Service 1988, 1993). It is useful to remember that Medicaid pioneered the use of prospective payment for hospitals long before Medicare's adoption of the system.

Two important variants of hospital payment systems, permitted by waiver authority, are all-payer systems and selective contracting. In the all-payer system used by Maryland, Medicaid pays a rate similar to that of private insurers, as established by a rate-setting board or similar body. The payment level usually includes an assessment to help pay hospitals with high uncompensated care costs. In selective contracting, used by California and parts of Washington, hospitals compete with each other to get contracts to provide Medicaid services. In 1991, California's average inpatient cost per enrollee was about two-thirds the national average (Johns 1989, Holahan 1988). Other hospital cost-containment systems that grew during the decade were utilization control or review, including upper limits on reimbursable inpatient days per year or per spell of illness, preadmission approval, and similar methods. About two-thirds of the states now have such controls (Congressional Research Service 1993).

PHYSICIAN, LABORATORY, AND RADIOLOGY SERVICES

Physician, laboratory, and radiology services comprise the third largest acute care service category, costing $7.4 billion in 1992. As shown in table 7.4, physician service expenditures per enrollee grew slightly faster than the rate of inflation for adults, children, and the blind and disabled in both 1984–90 and 1990–92. The overall constant dollar expenditure per enrollee grew somewhat more quickly (5.4 percent per year) in 1990–92 than in 1984–90 (2.6 percent per year). For the elderly, however, constant dollar physician expenditures per enrollee fell slightly in 1984–90. This is probably because the growth among QMB and dually enrolled Medicaid-Medicare aged led to smaller increases in elderly expenditures than in elderly enrollment, as previously described.

One reason why physician expenditures per enrollee have risen is that many states increased physician payment rates. Many of these were selective increases, targeting primary care, obstetric, and pediatric services, and were designed to increase physician participation in Medicaid. A longstanding complaint has been that most states

Table 7.4 PHYSICIAN/LABORATORY AND RADIOLOGY: MEDICAID EXPENDITURES BY ELIGIBILITY GROUP

| | Expenditures ($ 1992) | | | Expenditures per Enrollee ($ 1992) | | | | |
| | Level ($) | | Average Annual Change (%) | | Level ($) | | Average Annual Change (%) | | Share of Expenditures in 1992 (%) |
Eligibility Group	1984 (millions)	1992 (millions)	1984–90	1990–92	1984	1992	1984–90	1990–92	
All enrollees	4,035	7,358	4.8	17.5	161.13	208.50	2.6	5.4	100.0
Adult enrollees	1,358	2,661	6.5	15.8	230.23	322.56	4.3	4.3	36.2
Child enrollees	1,205	2,345	4.9	20.8	94.87	127.08	2.8	6.6	31.9
Aged enrollees	471	467	−4.3	13.6	143.64	124.14	−4.9	7.9	6.3
Blind and disabled enrollees	1,001	1,885	5.5	16.9	316.21	390.64	1.5	6.1	25.6

Note: Arizona and U.S. territories are not included.

have relatively low Medicaid payment rates to physicians, which reduce physician participation. In 1990 Medicaid physician fees for the nonelderly averaged 65 percent of private fees, 74 percent of Medicare prevailing charges, and 85 percent of Medicare allowed charges, even though there was considerable variation among states (Holahan 1991). Although it is commonly claimed that Medicaid's physician payment rates are low, they are actually comparable to, and often higher than, physician fees paid in Canada (Welch, Katz, and Zuckerman 1992). Although there has been concern about the adequacy of physician payments in general, recent policies have especially encouraged states to raise obstetric and pediatric payment rates to increase access. Medicaid obstetric and primary care services were relatively better paid than hospital visits or laboratory tests, when compared to other payers. Many states increased obstetric payment rates in 1990, spurred by changes in OBRA 89.[6]

Although Medicaid is often criticized for paying physicians poorly, the program pioneered physician payment reforms during the 1980s. Before Medicare adopted a relative value scale (RVS) system of paying physicians, several Medicaid states had already adopted physician fee schedules, most notably California's RVS system. In 1987, 31 states used physician fee schedules; this number rose to 42 by 1989. The rest of the states used systems based on prevailing charges, akin to the old Medicare system and most private health insurance.

OUTPATIENT HOSPITAL AND CLINIC SERVICES

Even though outpatient hospital and clinic services are fundamental to Medicaid, they have often been targets of criticism. Many Medicaid clients use emergency rooms or other outpatient clinics because they have no routine physician or source of medical care. For example, it was recently estimated that one-half to two-thirds of Medicaid emergency room visits were for nonemergency problems (Office of the Inspector General, U.S. Department of Health and Human Services 1992). Excessive use of outpatient services is of concern because of cost and quality issues. Outpatient payments for a given procedure are generally higher than an equivalent payment for a physician office visit, since the outpatient payments generally include higher institutional costs. Moreover, quality may be worse, since it is more difficult to assure continuity of physician-patient relations in outpatient settings, especially emergency rooms. One study found that use of outpatient hospital services was highest in areas with low Medicaid physician reimbursement rates, suggesting that use of outpatient care may be a reflection of poor access to private physicians (Cohen 1989)

During the past decade, outpatient costs have been one of the fastest growing services in Medicaid. As seen in table 7.5, outpatient hospital expenditures rose rapidly: constant dollar expenditures per enrollee grew an average of 7.4 percent per year during 1984–90 and 12.1 percent per year for 1990–92. Since outpatient services do not earn DSH payments, it is clear that outpatient services showed a more sustained and higher *real* growth rate than inpatient services. Prior analyses (Reilly, Clauser and Baugh 1990) have indicated that most of the increase in Medicaid outpatient costs between 1982 to 1988 was explained by increases in the number of recipients (service users). On a more modest level, the increase was the result of changes in average payment per recipient. In other words, increasing service use has been the major contributor to rising outpatient costs.

Unlike inpatient and physician expenditures, Medicaid outpatient expenditures per aged enrollee grew. This is somewhat puzzling, since outpatient services are also covered by Medicare, so that we expected declines paralleling those for inpatient and physician costs per enrollee. A plausible explanation of this paradox is that the implementation of the Medicare prospective payment system, as well as other changes in medical practice patterns and technology, led hospitals to shift care from inpatient to outpatient settings. Even though Medicare was paying much of the costs for the outpatient care, the increasing use of outpatient services also meant greater Medicaid payments in terms of deductibles and copayments.

Another trend that increased outpatient costs during this period was the shifting of the costs of maternal and child health services from state-funded programs to Medicaid, in order to earn more matching dollars. This would have increased both clinic and physician expenditures borne by Medicaid. As discussed in chapter 5, many states deliberately tried to shift maternal and child health services under the Medicaid umbrella.

States have instituted many changes in payment methods for outpatient care in recent years. For example, states have tended to shift from retrospective payment to prospective payment systems. Between 1987 and 1989, the number of states using prospective payment systems rose from 9 to 29 (Intergovernmental Health Policy Project 1989).

A final policy change for outpatient services was the development

Table 7.5 HOSPITAL OUTPATIENT AND CLINIC: MEDICAID EXPENDITURES BY ELIGIBILITY GROUP

Eligibility Group	Expenditures ($ 1992)			Expenditures per Enrollee ($ 1992)				
	Level ($)		Average Annual Change (%)	Level ($)		Average Annual Change (%)		Share of Expenditures in 1992 (%)
	1984 (millions)	1992 (millions)	1984–90	1990–92	1984	1992	1984–90	1990–92	
All enrollees	2,918	7,919	9.7	24.9	116.52	224.37	7.4	12.1	100.0
Adult enrollees	791	1,938	7.6	25.8	134.13	234.90	5.3	13.3	24.5
Child enrollees	953	2,398	7.3	28.5	75.02	129.91	5.1	13.4	30.3
Aged enrollees	196	463	7.9	22.3	59.77	123.14	7.3	16.2	5.8
Blind and disabled enrollees	978	3,120	13.5	22.3	308.85	646.52	9.2	11.1	39.4

Note: Arizona and U.S. territories are not included.

of Federally Qualified Health Center (FQHC) status. FQHC status is given to clinics that receive federal funds as a community or migrant health center or a health center for the homeless. FQHC status is also given to some similar, "look-alike" centers. FQHCs must be paid 100 percent of their reasonable costs. This affected about 700 federally funded centers and a smaller number of "look-alikes." This policy was developed to ensure that Medicaid was covering its costs in these centers for medically underserved areas or populations. Preliminary findings indicate that FQHC status has led to substantial revenue increases for community health centers (Lewis-Idema et al. 1992).

PRESCRIPTION DRUGS

Although prescription drugs are an optional service, most states (38) offered drug coverage to all enrollees in 1991. Another 16 states offered drug coverage to categorically eligible enrollees (for example, AFDC and SSI recipients, but not medically needy). Drug expenditures are very unevenly distributed across the four eligibility groups—adults, children, aged, and blind and disabled. As shown in table 7.6, average annual expenditures per aged, blind, or disabled enrollee are roughly 6 times higher than for adults and about 13 times higher than for children. This conforms to the belief that aged and disabled clients have far greater chronic medical problems that require medication. Since Medicare does not cover prescription drugs, the costs for the aged reflect the full cost of providing drugs for the elderly.

Since 1984 the changes in drug expenditures per enrollee have been modest, after adjusting for inflation in retail drug prices. During 1984–90 drug prices rose 3.5 percent per year faster than inflation and actually fell 4.4 percent per year from 1990 to 1992 (table 7.6). Much of that decline may have been caused by changes in drug payment policies. OBRA 90 required that pharmaceutical companies provide rebates for prescription drugs to state Medicaid programs after January 1, 1991. The policy goal was that Medicaid, as a major purchaser of prescription drugs, should get volume discounts on prices. The rebate program required a 10 percent discount on multiple-source (that is, generic) drugs. For single-source or some "innovator" drugs, the rebates are based on the "best price" offered by the manufacturer to volume purchasers. In 1992, the level of drug rebates collected was $900 million. Since some drug prices may have

Table 7.6 PRESCRIPTION DRUGS: MEDICAID EXPENDITURES BY ELIGIBILITY GROUP

Eligibility Group	Expenditures ($ 1992)			Expenditures per Enrollee ($ 1992)				
	Level ($)		Average Annual Change (%)	Level ($)		Average Annual Change (%)		Share of Expenditures in 1992 (%)
	1984 (millions)	1992 (millions)	1984–90	1990–92	1984	1992	1984–90	1990–92	
All enrollees	3,935	6,216	5.7	6.5	157.15	176.14	3.5	-4.4	100.0
Adult enrollees	612	748	2.5	2.7	103.76	90.67	0.3	-7.5	12.0
Child enrollees	427	774	5.5	14.6	33.60	41.95	3.4	1.1	12.5
Aged enrollees	1,518	2,006	3.5	3.6	462.82	533.22	2.9	-1.6	32.3
Blind and disabled enrollees	1,379	2,689	9.0	7.8	435.47	557.08	4.9	-2.1	43.2

Note: Arizona and U.S. territories are not included.

increased owing to the drug rebate policies, the amount collected is not necessarily equivalent to the level of savings.

Although the rebate program saved some money, some states believed that they lost money owing to a related requirement that states have "open formularies." A formulary is the list of drugs that are approved for coverage. Some states had closed formularies and did not cover certain drugs—for example, high price drugs or drugs with a cheaper substitute. The open formulary requirement meant that states had to cover virtually all marketed drugs (excluding experimental drugs). In some cases, this may have increased costs.

Although drugs are an optional service and a relatively expensive one ($6.2 billion in 1992), states did not make major cutbacks in their drug programs. Instead of major reductions in drug benefits, states engaged in a variety of incremental reforms, such as the rebate initiatives mentioned above. Another common change was to require small copayments (for example, $1 per prescription) and to reduce payments to pharmacists by that level. Some states developed more rigorous procedures than the federal rebate program to help contain costs.

EARLY AND PERIODIC SCREENING, DIAGNOSTIC AND TREATMENT

Early and Periodic Screening, Diagnostic, and Treatment services were designed to serve as the prevention and screening component of Medicaid for child health, including vision, hearing, and dental health and developmental disabilities. States have long been required to provide periodic screening services for children under age 21 and to treat the disorders detected during screenings. However, EPSDT has often been considered problematic owing to poor implementation and participation. One of the problems was that a relatively low share of eligible children were participating. In 1989, 39 percent of eligible children were estimated to participate. OBRA 89 established the goal that all states reach 80 percent participation by 1995 and also required reporting. In addition, the law expanded EPSDT by requiring states to provide testing whenever a child is suspected of having a problem, not just at periodic intervals. More important, it required that Medicaid pay for treatment of problems detected, even if it does not otherwise cover those services.

As shown in table 7.7, the constant dollar costs of EPSDT per child enrollee rose much more rapidly during 1990–92 (23.7 percent per year) than during 1984–90 (2.6 percent per year). This suggests that the recent policy initiatives greatly spurred expansion of EPSDT. Even so, EPSDT is a relatively small and inexpensive program, costing a total of $432 million in 1992, or about $23 per child enrollee.

MEDICARE PAYMENTS

Medicaid serves as a wraparound to Medicare for many low-income elderly persons (and to some disabled persons who are eligible for Medicare). For QMBs, Medicaid pays for Medicare premiums, deductibles, and copayments that the elderly would otherwise have to bear out-of-pocket. States may, if they like, also provide QMBs with additional Medicaid services, such as drugs or nursing home care. For elderly who are otherwise eligible for Medicare, such as SSI recipients, the state can pay Medicare premiums, deductibles, and copayments in lieu of paying for these services just through Medicaid. In these instances, Medicaid serves as the payer of last resort and, beyond the deductibles and copayments, only pays for services not covered by Medicare, such as prescription drugs or nursing home care. Medicaid payments to Medicare grew rapidly between 1984 and 1992 (table 7.7).[7] By 1992, Medicaid spent $2.3 billion on Medicare payments, or $617 per elderly enrollee. This reflects the growth of QMBs since 1988, as well as dually enrolled Medicaid-Medicare aged, as discussed earlier.

MANAGED CARE, HMOs, AND GROUP HEALTH

One of the most important trends in Medicaid is the growing use of HMOs and other managed care. Managed care includes "regular" HMOs and primary care case management (PCCM). HMO payments are based on a fixed, capitated payment per enrollee. In primary care case management (PCCM), a primary care physician serves as a gatekeeper to other medical or surgical care, but visits are usually still paid on a fee-for-service basis. However, the data reported in table 7.7 only encompass HMO-type costs, not fee-for-service costs incurred among PCCM clients. HMO expenditures (in constant dol-

Table 7.7 EPSDT AND PAYMENTS TO MEDICARE AND HMOs: MEDICAID EXPENDITURES BY ELIGIBILITY GROUP

Eligibility Group	Expenditures ($ 1992)				Expenditures per Enrollee ($ 1992)			
	Level ($)		Average Annual Change (%)		Level ($)		Average Annual Change (%)	
	1984 (millions)	1992 (millions)	1984–90	1990–92	1984	1992	1984–90	1990–92
EPSDT	166	432	4.7	40.2	13.09	23.39	2.6	23.7
Medicare payment	728	2,320	13.2	23.1	222.15	616.83	12.5	17.0
HMO payment	647	2,559	17.9	21.2	25.85	72.50	15.5	8.8

Notes: For EPSDT, expenditures are per child enrollee. "Medicare payment" is for elderly enrollees only. "HMO payment" includes all enrollees. Arizona and U.S. territories are not included.

lars) per enrollee grew 15.5 percent per year between 1984 and 1990 and another 8.8 percent per year between 1990 and 1992 (table 7.7). HCFA-2082 data do not show the number of HMO enrollees, the distribution of expenditures by age category, or the number of persons actually enrolled in managed care plans. Since a substantial share of Medicaid managed care involves a PCCM fee-for-service system, the HMO and group health payments understate the total level of managed care in Medicaid. The number of Medicaid recipients in managed care plans has been reported to rise from 2 percent in 1982 to 12 percent in 1992 (Intergovernmental Health Policy Project 1993b). In the past several years, growth has been particularly rapid in the PCCM plans, since they can be more readily developed within existing networks of physicians.

In 1992, 36 states had one or more managed care programs, and another 13 states plan to have them by 1994 (U.S. General Accounting Office 1993). The managed care programs always target AFDC-type participants, although some states also include disabled or aged participants. One important shift is that programs are increasingly becoming mandatory for some clients (for example, all AFDC participants in a certain area); 26 states had at least one mandatory managed care program. Mandatory programs, which require HCFA approval for a freedom-of-choice waiver, are used to ensure a sufficiently large number of managed care clients (to make them attractive to managed care plans) and to avoid selective enrollment of healthier persons (to help avoid "skimming"). Further, since Medicaid services are free to enrollees, they have little incentive to volunteer to join managed care plans. The most singular example of Medicaid managed care is the Arizona Health Care Cost Containment System (AHCCCS), a mandatory statewide capitated plan. AHCCCS was created in 1982 under a waiver as a substitute for Medicaid; before its initiation, Arizona had no Medicaid program at all. Arizona recently began a capitated long-term care plan also.

Although managed care has grown rapidly in recent years, Medicaid clients are still enrolled in managed care much less than the general population; roughly 15 percent of the general population was in HMOs and another 15 percent were in preferred provider organizations (PPOs) in 1991 (Health Insurance Association of America 1992). During the early 1980s, Medicaid managed care grew slowly because it was difficult to enroll clients or providers into voluntary managed care plans and because of some early scandals. However, in recent years, Medicaid managed care has accelerated rapidly, as states have begun to develop more PCCM plans and more mandatory managed care plans.

Previous research about Medicaid managed care has yielded mixed results. Common findings are that managed care is associated with increased access to medical care and reduced use of outpatient hospital care, especially emergency room use (Hurley, Freund, and Paul 1993; Miller and Gengler, forthcoming; and Wade 1993). Because managed care plans direct enrollees to specific physicians or medical providers, they know where to get routine care. This increases overall utilization of medical services, but reduces their use of outpatient care.

Findings differ about whether managed care reduces inpatient hospital use or overall medical expenditures per beneficiary. Some researchers have found reductions in inpatient use and in overall medical costs, whereas others have not. In their synthesis of studies of 25 programs, Hurley et al. (1993) estimated that savings in the range of 5 percent to 15 percent per beneficiary are reasonable, primarily owing to reductions in inpatient utilization. Although results are mixed about whether Medicaid managed care saves money, it is reasonable to say that, at best, savings are modest. One reason for this is that Medicaid fee-for-service payments are usually low (and as a result, access may also be low), so that minimal savings can be realized by Medicaid.

In discussing plans for expansion of Medicaid managed care, state officials have usually anticipated that managed care might save very modest amounts, such as 5 percent to 10 percent of acute care costs per enrollee (Holahan et al. 1992). Nonetheless, they have generally hoped that a shift to managed care would also improve program access and quality. In contrast, many advocates for low-income families worry about the implications of Medicaid managed care, especially of mandatory plans. They warn that managed care might result in underservice or poor quality care (Kosterlitz 1992).

OTHER ACUTE AND PREVENTIVE SERVICES

"Other" services include mandatory services, such as family planning, as well as optional services, such as dental, optometric, podiatric, and chiropractic services and transportation. Although these are relatively small services individually, together they totaled $5.2 billion in 1992, or about $148 per enrollee (table 7.8). As shown in the table, the expenditures per enrollee for "other" services usually grew less than the services discussed earlier. Possible reasons include: these smaller services had lower payment increases permitted by states, utilization grew less steeply, and states may have eliminated or trimmed these smaller services during budget cutting, especially in the 1990s.

SUMMARY

Beginning in the late 1980s, acute and preventive services became a larger share of Medicaid expenditures, reversing the previous trend in which long-term care was growing faster. The main reasons for this reversal were the development of DSH programs for inpatient care and the declining share of the program held by the aged, who dominate long-term care expenditures.

Another important trend included broad efforts to upgrade maternal and child health care. Along with the expansions of eligibility for pregnant women, many state Medicaid programs began to provide enhanced services to pregnant women, including services such as case management, risk assessment, nutritional or psychosocial counseling, and home visits. State Medicaid programs often worked with state maternal and child health staff to develop better packages of prenatal and perinatal care (Dubay et al. 1993).

In most cases, Medicaid expenditures per enrollee were growing more rapidly than the rate of inflation, highlighting the difficulties in controlling Medicaid costs. Hospital inpatient expenditures grew especially fast from 1990 to 1992, but this was almost entirely due to DSH payments. The area with the most rapid real growth in expenditures was outpatient hospital and clinic services.

Although these costs were escalating, federal and state Medicaid policymakers were undertaking a variety of initiatives to slow the rate of cost increases for acute and preventive care. There were important changes in the way that Medicaid pays for hospital (inpatient and outpatient) and physician services and for drugs. In addition to changes in how medical care is paid for, states were also experimenting with changes in how care is delivered to clients. Managed care is becoming a more important mode of providing acute and preventive services in the Medicaid program, especially for nondisabled adults

Table 7.8 OTHER ACUTE AND PREVENTIVE CARE: MEDICAID EXPENDITURES BY ELIGIBILITY GROUP

| | Expenditures ($ 1992) | | | | Expenditures per Enrollee ($ 1992) | | | | |
| | Level ($) | | Average Annual Change (%) | | Level ($) | | Average Annual Change ($) | | Share of Expenditures in 1992 (%) |
Eligibility Group	1984 (millions)	1992 (millions)	1984–90	1990–92	1984	1992	1984–90	1990–92	
All enrollees	2,628	5,217	5.7	19.2	104.94	147.81	3.5	7.0	100.0
Adult enrollees	699	1,153	1.3	23.5	118.45	139.79	−0.8	11.2	22.1
Child enrollees	730	1,479	5.6	20.8	57.47	80.12	3.5	6.5	28.3
Aged enrollees	401	626	5.0	8.0	122.32	166.43	4.3	2.7	12.0
Blind and disabled enrollees	799	1,959	9.3	19.8	252.14	405.87	5.3	8.8	37.5

Note: Arizona and U.S. territories are not included.

and children. State officials hope that managed care can improve patient access and help control spending increases.

Notes

1. Hospitals contend that Medicaid payments are usually less than the costs of treating patients; an American Hospital Association (1992) analysis suggested that hospitals lost $5 billion nationwide providing care to Medicaid patients in 1991 (including both inpatient and outpatient care).

2. We assumed that 13.2 percent of DSH payments and special revenues were for mental health in 1992 and that there were no mental health DSH payments in 1990. The 1992 percentages for mental health and inpatient services were computed based on discrepancies between HCFA-2082 and HCFA-64 levels because it appeared that DSH payments (which were often lump-sum payments) were the main source of discrepancy.

3. Expenditure growth per enrollee greater than the rate of inflation indicates that utilization is increasing, that services are becoming more intensive, and/or that reimbursements are rising faster than the rate of inflation. Aside from the DSH payments (which are essentially reimbursement rate increases), utilization and service intensity increases are the most likely explanations. These might occur because many of the new enrollees had active medical problems, such as pregnancy or AIDS.

4. DSH payments involve, first, a formula that determines which hospitals are called DSH hospitals and, second, a formula that determines the level of payment to each DSH hospital. These formulae typically include the volume of care provided both to Medicaid and uncompensated care.

5. For example, a county provides $10 million in an intergovernmental transfer to the state, and the county hospital gets $15 million in DSH payments. The county reduces its subsidy to the hospital by $13 million, so that the hospital has a net gain of $2 million and the county has a net gain of $3 million.

6. OBRA 89 encouraged states to increase obstetrician's payments and required more monitoring of participation rates by obstetricians.

7. In contrast to most of the data reported, Medicare payments and HMO payments are not listed on the HCFA-2082 and are drawn exclusively from the HCFA-64 data. One important implication is that these data do not reveal the number of or eligibility status of people who are enrolled to receive Medicare payments or HMO capitated payments. Thus, the estimates of the expenditures per enrollee are based on the overall number of people enrolled, assuming that Medicare-Medicaid dual enrollees are all elderly, although some are also disabled.

8. HMO payments are based on a fixed, capitated payment per enrollee. In primary care case management (PCCM), a primary care physician serves as a gatekeeper to other medical or surgical care, but visits are usually still paid on a fee-for-service basis.

Chapter Eight

CONCLUSIONS AND HEALTH CARE REFORM

The past decade was turbulent for Medicaid. In addition to tremendous growth, the program was constantly changing in response to both federal and state policy directives. During the early 1980s, Medicaid was cut back because of legislation enacted at the start of the Reagan administration. By the mid-1980s, Medicaid had resumed a cautious level of growth.

During the late 1980s, Medicaid underwent a series of policy changes that, in conjunction with the recession of the early 1990s, caused unprecedented growth in program enrollment and expenditures. These policy changes were set in motion in the mid-1980s as Congress, with encouragement from the states, passed a series of incremental expansions in program eligibility, especially aimed at pregnant women and children and the low-income elderly. Initially, the expansions were optional, but within a relatively short time most became mandatory.

Although the states initially supported the expansions, financing them became increasingly difficult for the states. Just as the mandates were being implemented, the nation entered a recession, which caused state revenues to decline precipitously. States, in other words, were being required to greatly expand their Medicaid programs while facing broad financial problems. The states responded to this situation by formally asking Congress for a moratorium on further Medicaid expansions. They also responded by rapidly developing new and controversial financing programs, such as provider tax and donation programs, and disproportionate-share (DSH) programs. Effectively, these programs shifted more of the cost of Medicaid to the federal government, which caused considerable alarm among federal policymakers. After protracted negotiations, a 1991 federal law was passed that sharply restricted states' use of special financing programs to pay for Medicaid. This series of events has caused increased tensions between states and the federal government over the Medicaid program.

This final chapter summarizes our examination of the Medicaid program over the last decade. We then discuss how Medicaid fits into health care reform proposals currently being undertaken or debated on both the state and national levels.

HIGHLIGHTS OF MAJOR FINDINGS

Program Eligibility

Eligibility for Medicaid underwent several major changes between 1981 and 1992. One of the most prominent of these was the eligibility expansions directed at pregnant women and children. Enacted out of concern over high infant mortality rates and eroding health care coverage of poor children, a series of federally mandated expansions of Medicaid targeted at pregnant women and children was adopted beginning in 1984. By 1992, states were required to extend Medicaid coverage to children under age 9 who live below the federal poverty line and to pregnant women below 133 percent of the poverty line. States also must phase in coverage to all children under age 19 with incomes below the federal poverty level. By the year 2002, all poor children will be covered by Medicaid.

By expressly tying Medicaid protection to the poverty line, these new eligibility expansions set national minimum income eligibility standards for pregnant women and children, much like those used for the SSI program. The expansions also greatly weakened the program's longstanding link with the AFDC program, reducing the state-to-state variation in eligibility.

Medicaid's link to another cash welfare program—the SSI program—was also loosened in the 1980s by the passage of the Qualified Medicare Beneficiaries mandates. These mandates required states to pay for Medicare cost sharing for Medicare beneficiaries with incomes up to 120 percent of the poverty line. Collectively, the federal mandates of the 1980s have reduced the fraction of Medicaid enrollees who also receive cash assistance, from 80 percent in 1984 to 60 percent in 1992.

Beyond breaking the historical link between cash welfare programs and Medicaid, the mandates also opened eligibility to whole new populations such as legalized aliens and the homeless. Thus, the eligibility expansions not only improved program access for many of the traditional Medicaid populations but also extended first-time access to others.

The precise impact of the eligibility expansions on health outcomes is at present not known. Although it is still too early to accurately measure the full effect of the mandates, preliminary studies on the impact of the pregnant women mandates suggest that although enrollment has been successful, no significant improvements in birth outcomes (such as reductions in infant mortality and in low birthweight) have been observed.

One consequence of the eligibility expansions is that more people receive health care coverage through Medicaid. Program enrollment has grown rapidly, particularly in recent years: between 1988 and 1992, Medicaid enrollment expanded from 25.4 million to 35.3 million, an increase of 10 million persons. The bulk of this growth, about half, can be attributed to newly entitled pregnant women and children.

Data from the Current Population Surveys demonstrate that, between 1988 and 1991, Medicaid enrolled a larger share of children, adult women, the aged, and the disabled, and that these increases occurred both among poor and near-poor individuals. Even though Medicaid coverage expanded, the proportion of the population without health insurance rose over that time period, as a result of declining employer-based health care coverage. Although Medicaid was serving more people all the time, its expansion did not keep pace with eroding employer-based insurance occurring because of broader national changes. However, the number of persons and the proportion of the population who lacked health care insurance would have been higher still had Medicaid not expanded as rapidly as it did. Thus, the Medicaid expansions in effect masked the decline in employer-related coverage.

The Medicaid expansions also contributed to a significant reduction in the inequality of Medicaid coverage among states that occurred throughout the 1980s: between 1979 and 1991 interstate differences in Medicaid coverage, measured relative to the poverty population, fell by about one-half. In the early part of that period, coverage variation among the states shrank as more generous states trimmed Medicaid eligibility both in response to the 1980–81 recession and OBRA 1981, which, among other things, reduced eligibility for welfare benefits. Interstate differences continued to decline in the mid- and late-1980s as less generous states increased Medicaid protection, largely in response to the pregnant women and children mandates.

Program Payment, Services, and Delivery

The Medicaid program also underwent significant changes in the way services were paid and delivered as well as the types of services covered. The principal goal of these changes was to control program costs by improving efficiency, adopting preventive services, or replacing higher-cost services with lower-cost ones. Through these changes, states served an important role as laboratories in which new health care policies were developed and tested. They also became more sophisticated health care purchasers.

Regarding payment changes, throughout the 1980s state Medicaid programs pioneered prospective payment systems for hospitals and physicians, which were subsequently adapted for use in Medicare. They also developed prospective payment systems for outpatient hospital services and nursing homes. More recently, 1990 federal legislation established the drug rebate system, a new approach to using volume purchasing power to reduce the purchase price of prescription drugs. These payment changes were designed to decrease costs while preserving Medicaid eligibility and benefit structures.

In some cases, Medicaid programs also altered the types of health care services provided. Three of the most prominent areas in which this occurred were: long-term care, maternal and child health care, and managed care. Regarding the first, over the decade states increasingly emphasized the use of home and community-based services as a lower-cost substitute for institutional care. Between 1984 and 1992, spending for home and community-based care grew twice as fast as that for institutional care. Most of this increased spending was for waiver programs that offer specific services for specialized populations, primarily the disabled and aged. Despite the rapid growth, expenditures for home and community-based care still comprise only about 10 percent of total long-term care expenditures.

Paralleling the expansions in eligibility for pregnant women and children were efforts to upgrade the quality of maternal and child health care. Payment levels for obstetricians and pediatricians were increased to encourage physician participation in the Medicaid program. Most states created enhanced packages of prenatal care services, including risk assessment, case management, nutritional and psychosocial services, and home visiting. In many cases state Medicaid programs worked closely with public health agencies to develop better systems of care. More recently, legislation was passed requiring states to strengthen EPSDT, the preventive health program for children.

For most of the decade, Medicaid lagged behind private insurance in the use of managed care, principally because several states had less-than-successful experiences with managed care in the early 1970s. In the past few years, however, Medicaid managed care plans have grown rapidly. In 1992, 12 percent of Medicaid recipients were enrolled in such plans, up from 2 percent in 1982. A growing trend has been the adoption of mandatory managed care plans for AFDC-type enrollees; previously, states had only voluntary plans. States hope that managed care will improve access for enrollees while controlling costs. Critics of Medicaid involvement in managed care, however, fear that quality of care will be reduced, especially under mandatory plans.

Over the last decade states have also made adjustments to provider payment levels, a particularly thorny issue for Medicaid. Medicaid has historically been viewed as paying providers poorly, which has discouraged physicians and nursing homes from participating in the program. Low Medicaid payment levels have also caused hospitals to shift costs to private pay patients. Important changes occurred during the late 1980s, however, that have boosted Medicaid payment levels. The Boren Amendment became a legal tool that hospitals and nursing homes used to formally challenge the adequacy of Medicaid reimbursement in courts. In addition, the rapid development of disproportionate-share programs provided windfalls to hospitals, especially public hospitals and other hospitals that served disproportionate shares of poor patients. In most states, these DSH windfalls also helped pay for care to uninsured patients. Finally, Congress, as part of OBRA 1989, required states to raise physician reimbursement for pediatricians and obstetricians. Because of the way Medicaid reimburses doctors, this increase most likely brought about increases for other physicians.

Program Expenditures and Financing

Mirroring the changes in program eligibility, payment, and services, Medicaid expenditure patterns have also changed dramatically over the past decade. Most notable is the recent rapid acceleration in Medicaid spending. Following moderate spending growth of about 10 percent per year throughout most of the 1980s, Medicaid spending began to surge in 1988. Program expenditures between 1988 and 1992 rose from $51.3 billion to nearly $113 billion, an average annual growth rate of 21.7 percent (nominal dollars). The major determinants of this sharp rise include enrollment increases caused by the recession and the federal mandates; increases in medical care prices; the federally mandated service expansions; and increases in utilization and costs above inflation.

Using a model that decomposed expenditure increases between 1988 and 1992, we found that growth in the number of recipients accounted for 36 percent of the increase, medical price inflation accounted for about 26 percent, and utilization and reimbursement above inflation accounted for 33 percent. Much of the increase in the last category was brought about by states' increasing use of special financing programs.

Beginning around 1989, state Medicaid programs were squeezed by two opposing forces: declining state revenues (due to the economic recession) and rising Medicaid costs (caused partly by the new federal mandates). Most states responded to this situation by establishing special financing programs, including using "special revenues" (from provider taxes and donations, and intergovernmental transfers) and expenditures in the form of disproportionate-share hospital payments. These programs, virtually nonexistent in the mid-1980s, exploded in size between 1990 and 1992. By 1992, $7.8 billion was collected in provider taxes and donations, and intergovernmental transfers and DSH payments reached $17.4 billion. When DSH payments are treated as a separate growth factor in the decomposition model, such payments account for nearly 26 percent of the total expenditure increase between 1988 and 1992. DSH payments, in other words, contributed almost as much to Medicaid expenditure growth over the 1988–92 period as did increases in the number of program recipients, and amounted to more than overall medical price inflation.

One consequence of states' use of special financing programs is that the federal government is now paying for a greater share of Medicaid costs. If the value of provider taxes, donations, and intergovernmental transfers is omitted (because these programs do not reflect true spending), then the federal share of Medicaid expenditures rises from 57.4 percent to 61.6 percent. However, despite the fact that special financing programs enabled states to leverage greater federal contributions to Medicaid, state spending rose sharply in recent years. Between 1990 and 1992, state Medicaid spending, including special revenues, increased on average 27 percent each year. Even if special revenues are netted out, state spending rose 17 percent per year (nominal dollars), a growth rate that has not been observed since the late 1970s.

Another consequence of special financing programs is that intergovernmental relations between states and the federal government became increasingly strained. The federal government viewed many of these programs as being inappropriate, and sought to have them outlawed as early as 1988. States, however, maintained that the federal government had no statutory authority to evaluate state sources of revenue for Medicaid. Moreover, the states argued that they needed special financing programs to pay for the unfunded federal mandates that they were being required to implement. Between 1988 and 1991, the Bush administration attempted several times to persuade Congress to regulate both provider tax and donation programs and DSH programs. Each time, however, the states managed to delay such regulation.

Finally, after prolonged negotiations between the administration and governors, Congress passed the Medicaid Voluntary Contributions and Provider-Specific Tax Amendments of 1991, which greatly limited the states' use of special financing programs. Key provisions include banning donations, requiring that provider taxes be "broad based," and capping total DSH payments. It appears that the new law, especially the DSH cap provision, has been effective in limiting expenditure increases. Preliminary data from federal fiscal year 1993 indicate that the Medicaid expenditure growth rate was 10 percent, less than half the 1992 rate (Health Care Financing Administration, Office of the Actuary, personal communication from John Klemm 1994).

Medicaid Problems and Gaps

Although much progress was made in improving the Medicaid program over the decade, many problems remain. One of the most important of these is that for many poor people, obtaining Medicaid eligibility has become increasingly difficult. Between 1980 and 1992, AFDC and medically needy income standards became more restrictive: after adjusting for the cost of living, qualifying income levels for AFDC recipients have generally declined by nearly 27 percent; and for the medically needy, nearly 30 percent. Poor nonpregnant women and persons with high medical costs thus have less access to Medicaid today than they did a decade ago.

Coupled with eroding eligibility is the persistence of interstate variation. Although program coverage became more similar across the country during the 1980s, it remains quite unequal. The average level of expenditures per recipients, once they are in Medicaid, remained almost as dissimilar in 1992 as it was in 1984. States continue to have wide disparities in generosity of benefits and payments to providers.

Perhaps a bigger concern is that many poor people continue to lack health insurance yet are ineligible for Medicaid, a problem that has plagued the program since its inception nearly three decades ago. Because of the categorical restrictions imposed by the program, some people (for example, males, childless couples, and childless nonpregnant women who are not disabled) do not qualify for Medicaid, no matter how poor they are. Consequently, in 1992 only about half of the poor were covered by Medicaid.

Even for those with Medicaid protection, gaining access to health care continues to pose difficulties. The limited number of doctors who participate in Medicaid reduces recipients' access to medical care. Only one-third of doctors fully participate in the program, another one-third restrict the number of Medicaid patients they see, and about one-quarter reject Medicaid patients all together (American Medical Association 1991). A major reason why doctors are reluctant to see Medicaid patients is low payment levels, which for a routine office visit average about 60 percent of the actual cost. Although it is more difficult for hospitals to refuse care, data from the American Hospital Association indicate that a small number of hospitals treat the bulk of Medicaid recipients while the rest treat very few.

To many analysts, the greatest problem has been the explosive growth in the cost of Medicaid, more than doubling between 1989 and 1992, in contrast to most of the 1980s, when Medicaid grew more slowly than either Medicare or private health care costs. The soaring cost of Medicaid has increased federal debt and caused states to hold down spending for other programs.

STATE HEALTH REFORM INITIATIVES AND MEDICAID

The problems of rapidly accelerating health care costs, especially for Medicaid, and the rising number of uninsured people, have led states to initiate health care reform. Virtually every state is considering or implementing some type of legislation that restructures their health care system (Intergovernmental Health Policy Project 1993c). The reform strategies vary significantly, ranging from incremental change (such as altering small group insurance regulations) to a complete overhaul of the health care system. Many states have already enacted major health reform measures, including Hawaii, Minnesota, Oregon, Tennessee, and Washington. Proposals are pending in other states, including Florida, Colorado, Georgia, Kentucky, New York, Vermont, West Virginia and Wisconsin.

States' approaches to health reform generally fall into two categories: those addressing health care financing and those addressing the delivery of services (Rogal and Helms 1993). Most often state efforts combine both financing and delivery efforts. States are contemplating a wide variety of financing reforms, ranging from flexible spending accounts (Oklahoma) to a Canadian-style, single-payer system (Vermont). Many states are also contemplating employing stricter cost controls, such as expenditure targets and community rating as part of their reforms.

Among the most noteworthy of the state health initiatives:

□   The Oregon Health Plan expands Medicaid eligibility to all state residents with incomes below the poverty line, but, as a trade-off, limits the types of medical services (based on a list of "prioritized" health services) covered by its Medicaid program. The plan also includes a "play or pay" employer mandate in which employers are required to either purchase insurance or pay into a state insurance pool. Although Oregon's "rationing" plan was approved by HCFA in early 1993, budgetary and political problems have clouded its implementation schedule.

□   By expanding the Medicaid program, Minnesota's Minnesota-Care program (applying the Medicaid option 1902(r)(2) provision that permits states to set enhanced income and asset thresholds) provides protection to all families with children whose incomes fall below 275 percent of poverty. In 1994, Minnesota will extend protection to all state residents who have been uninsured for four months and have not had access to employer-based insurance for 18 months.

□   Tennessee's TennCare program extends Medicaid coverage to all persons whose incomes fall below 100 percent of poverty. The state hopes to finance the expansion, at least in part, by enrolling all recipients into lower-cost managed care plans. Although it is too early to assess the plan which began January 1, 1994, there were early indications of implementation problems associated with provider concerns about low capitation rates.

□   The state of Washington has enacted a sweeping package of health care reforms. Under the Health Services Act, by 1999 all Washington residents must be covered by a certified health plan, which will offer a specified health service package. Universal coverage will be achieved through an employer mandate and significant expansions of Medicaid and Washington's program for the uninsured. Cost containment measures for the reform include premium caps and managed competition.

While publicity and debate surrounding national health care reform (discussed below) have overshadowed state reform efforts, it is important to bear in mind that several states have already made broad, ambitious changes in their health care systems and radical changes in their Medicaid programs. If a broad national health care reform law is passed, then state health reforms may serve as transitional phases prior to implementation of federal reforms or may be allowable alternatives to federal plans. In the absence of sweeping federal action, though, states will continue to lead health care reform efforts.

NATIONAL HEALTH CARE REFORM AND MEDICAID

More than 25 years after the nation last considered restructuring its health care system, health care reform has recently resurfaced as a national issue. The structure of the Medicaid program and assistance to low-income persons is a key issue in the reform debate. Should the program be replaced by national health reform or should Medicaid just be redesigned? Who among the poor should be covered under reform? What services should be provided? How should program costs be contained?

There are three basic approaches to reforming health care protection of the poor, all of which are embodied in one form or another in the many legislative proposals presently being considered by Congress. The most modest of the three reforms is to build on the existing system and simply expand Medicaid so that more low-income persons are covered. Broadening Medicaid is a major element of the Michel bill, the Affordable Health Care Now Act of 1993 (H.R. 3080).

Another strategy to reform health care coverage for the poor is to eliminate or significantly reduce the scope of Medicaid and enroll the poor (either all or most) in the private health insurance plans used by other Americans. Mainstreaming Medicaid recipients is a central feature of several health reform proposals, including President Clinton's Health Security Act (H.R. 3600/S. 1757), the Cooper/ Breaux Managed Competition Act of 1993 (H.R. 3222/S. 1579), and the Chafee/Thomas Health Equity and Access Reform Act of 1993 (S. 1770/H.R. 3704).

A third approach, the most sweeping of the three strategies, is to replace Medicaid altogether and fully merge it into a federally sponsored national health insurance plan that would cover the entire population. Such an approach, commonly referred to as the "single-payer" approach, is akin to the Canadian health care system which is sponsored and financed entirely by the government. The McDermott/ Wellstone American Health Security Act of 1993 (H.R. 1200/S. 491) is closely modelled after the Canadian system.

In sum, the current legislative strategies designed to improve the U.S. health care system are highly diverse. Thus, the proposals' effects on Medicaid vary widely. Some call for incremental changes to Medicaid whereas others call for wholesale replacement of the program. In table 8.1 we summarize key provisions of the alternative health reform proposals, especially as they relate to Medicaid and health care for low-income persons. Specifically, we assess each by the following criteria:

□ Breadth of coverage for the poor and near poor population;
□ Depth of service coverage and protection against out-of-pocket costs;
□ Strength of cost containment measures; and
□ Improvement in eligibility and financing inequities across the states.

It is important to remember that these legislative proposals are changing rapidly. Although the authors have sought to be as current as possible when describing these plans (as of January 1994), the proposals will undoubtedly evolve during legislative and public discussion and debate.

The Clinton Administration Proposal

The Clinton Administration's Health Security Act calls for universal health care coverage which will be achieved by employer and individual mandates. It relies on both managed competition and global budgets as cost containment measures. The plan would use *regional*

Table 8.1 SUMMARY ASSESSMENTS OF MAJOR NATIONAL HEALTH CARE REFORM PROPOSALS AS THEY RELATE TO
MEDICAID AND LOW-INCOME PERSONS AS OF JANUARY 1994

Proposal	Coverage of Poor and Near Poor	Services Covered and Out-of-Pocket Costs	Cost Containment	Equity Across States
Clinton Health Security Act	Covers all poor and non-poor through Medicaid, employer mandates and subsidies to low-income families. Subsidizes working families to 150% of poverty and nonworkers (who must also cover employer portion of premiums) to 250% of poverty with sliding scales. Persons on AFDC or SSI will still pay no premiums. Other Medicaid clients (e.g., expansion groups, medically needy) will have to pay premiums, depending on their income and employment status.	Integrates Medicaid acute and preventive services into regional health alliances. Relatively broad standard set of acute and preventive benefits. Most low-income clients will probably join mainstream managed care or other low-cost plans. Modest cost sharing. Medicaid retains long-term care services and mandates medically needy for nursing home benefits. Creates new state block grants for home and community-based services for severely disabled.	Limited managed competition among plans to reduce costs. There will also be limits on insurance premiums. In addition, there are limits on Medicaid and Medicare spending. Replaces DSH with much smaller vulnerable population adjustment.	Access to acute and preventive services will be more uniform across nation. There may be state differences for long-term care services. The state maintenance of effort provisions will cause historically generous states to provide more funding, regardless of current needs.

			For those below poverty, access should be similar across the nation. For 100–200% of poverty range, there may still be some differences due to voluntary nature of plan. There will be greater interstate differences in long-term care. Interstate financing for acute care should be more equitable.
Cooper/Breaux Managed Competition Act	Voluntary program to improve affordability of insurance. No individual or employer mandates. Federal government will subsidize insurance premiums for low-income: full subsidy for those under 100% of poverty and sliding assistance up to 200% of poverty.	Medicaid merged into health plan purchasing cooperatives. Standard benefit package for acute and preventive services, to be defined later. Drugs, vision, hearing aids covered for those under 100% of poverty. Cost sharing to be determined later. Long-term care gradually becomes solely a state responsibility.	Managed competition to reduce costs of health plans. No global budgets or premium limits. Eliminates Medicaid and DSH. Medicare spending limits.	
Chafee/Thomas Senate Republican Health Equity and Access Reform Act	Aims for universal coverage by 2005. But if Medicaid, Medicare and other savings are not attained, coverage of low-income may be delayed. For non-Medicaid low-income, federal subsidies to be phased in. Employers must offer, but need not pay for health insurance.	States have option to merge Medicaid into the health plans. Standard benefits package for health plan acute and preventive services to be determined later. Cost sharing to be determined later. Long-term services are not included.	Managed competition to reduce costs of health plans. No global budgets or premium limits. Reductions in Medicaid and Medicare spending growth to subsidize program. Phases DSH out.	Medicaid would still vary among states, but the subsidies for the low-income, if implemented, would be uniform. Because federal Medicaid payment per capita is capped, interstate Medicaid differences could become greater.

continued

Table 8.1 SUMMARY ASSESSMENTS OF MAJOR NATIONAL HEALTH CARE REFORM PROPOSALS AS THEY RELATE TO MEDICAID AND LOW-INCOME PERSONS AS OF JANUARY 1994 (continued)

Wellstone/McDermott American Health Security Act (Single Payer)	Universal coverage with no premiums for acute and preventive services. Premiums required for long-term care.	Integrates Medicaid into state health plans. Broad package of standard acute and preventive benefits, with no cost sharing. Long-term care for severely disabled included in program.	Costs contained through strict global budgeting. States can set physician fees, hospital and nursing home budgets. Eliminates Medicaid and DSH.	Access to acute, preventive and long-term care will be more uniform. States will contribute 15% of cost, but the formula for their contributions is not clear.
Michel House Republican Affordable Health Care Now Act	Voluntary program to improve affordability of health insurance. Permits states to offer coverage in health allowance plans up to 100% of poverty, with an option for buy-ins up to 200% of poverty. No individual or employer mandates.	States may create health allowance plans to offer private insurance to Medicaid clients. For health allowance plan buy-ins, cost sharing may be required. Permits states to establish purchasing cooperatives. No standard benefits packages under plans. Unclear if preventive or long-term care is covered.	Voluntary managed competition. No global budgets. Limits premium increases for small employers. States can use DSH funds to pay for extra costs of health allowance plan for low-income clients.	Permits states to expand health allowance plans to 100–200% of poverty. There might be more equity across states. Probably maintains historical differences in relative state effort and costs of Medicaid.

health alliances, geographically based institutions that would negotiate premium prices with a variety of health insurance companies to provide a standard benefit package. Within a given health alliance, contracts would be made with several insurers that would vary both in price and service delivery (for example, HMO or fee-for-service). Consumers would then choose among the various health care plans.

The intent behind the health alliances is to group enough consumers to ensure active competition among the various health care plans, thereby controlling costs. Costs would also be contained through global budgets which would cap both the level and rate of growth of health insurance premiums. Another cost containment feature of the Clinton proposal is that every American—regardless of income—will be required to bear some direct out-of-pocket expense for at least part of their health care.

Under the Health Security Act employers with fewer than 5,000 employees would make payments to the regional health alliances to cover 80 percent of the cost of the weighted average premium of all plans offered by the alliance. (Employees with more than 5,000 workers could join the regional alliance in their area or establish a corporate alliance; in either case, they are responsible for 80 percent of the insurance premium.) Families and individuals would pay the remainder of the cost, with the amount depending upon the plan selected. Self-employed individuals, nonworking persons, and Medicaid enrollees would also be enrolled in the regional health alliances. Depending upon their income, some of these individuals would be entitled to premium subsidies. Thus, in principle, all individuals in a given alliance—whether employed in a small or medium-sized firm, self-employed, unemployed, or enrolled in Medicaid—would have access to a variety of health plans, although the affordability of plans may vary.

Current Medicaid recipients would be enrolled in the health alliances through a variety of routes (table 8.2). Cash-assistance recipients (those in AFDC or SSI) who reside in a household with no employed worker would enroll through the Medicaid program. It is anticipated that most Medicaid recipients would join HMOs or low-cost sharing plans offered by the alliance in their local area. If a Medicaid recipient joins a plan whose cost was at or below the average premium within their health alliance, their premium would be fully subsidized by the plan. They would, however, be required to pay some copayments. Cash-assistance recipients who are employed (or live in a household with an employed worker) would

Table 8.2 HOW CURRENT MEDICAID RECIPIENTS WOULD BE COVERED FOR ACUTE AND PREVENTIVE HEALTH CARE UNDER THE CLINTON PROPOSAL, THE HEALTH SECURITY ACT

Type of Medicaid Recipient under Current System	Family Employment Status	Who Pays the Premiums	Premium	HMO Cost Sharing
Cash-assisted (AFDC or SSI)	Not employed	Medicaid	Fully subsidized if they join the plan at or below the average premium; otherwise partially subsidized.	$10 per office visit; $5 per drug prescription
Cash-assisted (AFDC or SSI)	Employed	Employer and Medicaid	Fully subsidized if they join the plan at or below the average premium; otherwise partially subsidized	$10 per office visit; $5 per drug prescription
Non-cash-assisted (for example, expansion groups or medically needy)	Employed	Employer and family	On a sliding scale, subsidies available for those with incomes up to 150 percent of poverty.	$10 per office visit; $5 per drug prescription
Non-cash-assisted (for example, expansion groups or medically needy)	Not employed	Family (as employer and employee)	On a sliding scale, subsidies available for those with incomes up to 250 percent of poverty.	$10 per office visit; $5 per drug prescription

Source: The Urban Institute, Washington, D.C.

be enrolled in the alliance by their employer. The employer would pay 80 percent of the cost of the weighted average plan, with subsidies for small, low-wage firms.

Non–cash-assistance recipients (for example, those covered under the pregnant women and children mandates) would no longer be covered by Medicaid. If they are employed they would be treated just like other employed persons: employers would pay 80 percent of the cost of the weighted average premium. Employees with incomes below 150 percent of poverty, regardless of prior Medicaid status, would be entitled to subsidies for the difference between the weighted average premium and the employer contribution.

Non–cash-assisted Medicaid recipients who are not employed would, in principle, be required to bear the full cost of the premium. This is the same general policy that would apply to other self-employed persons or unemployed persons not on Medicaid. Most of these individuals, however, will benefit from premium subsidies offered by the government to those with incomes below 250 percent of poverty.

Medicaid would still provide supplemental services that are not covered in the basic benefit plan. Most prominent among these services are institutional long-term care services such as nursing facility care, intermediate care facilities for the mentally retarded, and inpatient mental health care. Current Medicaid home- and community-based care would be provided in large part by the Home and Community Based Services program, a new federal program created under the Clinton plan. Thus, individuals who are presently receiving institutional care through the Medicaid program—and other specific services—would form the core of the residual Medicaid population. The residual Medicaid program, in other words, would be almost exclusively a long-term care program.

The Clinton health care proposal mandates state Medicaid programs to continue to make payments for covering cash-assisted recipients. States will be required to pay to the health alliance an amount equal to 95 percent of what they spent on health care per capita in the year prior to the implementation of the reform, adjusted forward for inflation. In addition, states would also be required to pay the alliance what they are currently paying for acute care services for non-cash-assisted recipients (for example, the newly mandated expansion groups and the medically needy), despite the fact that the Medicaid program will no longer be formally responsible for such recipients. These payments—which will go to the regional alliances—will be used to partially offset the cost of the various premium subsidies for low-income persons that are called for by the reform.

Measured against the four criteria in table 8.1, the Clinton Administration proposal does reasonably well. Since the plan calls for universal, mandatory health care coverage, the poor and the near-poor would be fully covered. Moreover, because the proposal specifies a rich package of acute and preventive services with modest cost-sharing, the health care needs of low-income persons should be well provided for. For the medically needy, the Clinton proposal expands protection by mandating that states provide medically needy coverage for long-term care services.

Inequities in Medicaid's coverage of the poor across states should be greatly reduced under the Clinton proposal. Since the plan would create a standard benefit package which would be provided to all Americans regardless of place of residence or income level, access to health care for the poor should become uniform across the states.

Health care access for the poor should also improve relative to individuals currently covered by private health insurance. A principal goal of the Clinton proposal is that low-income persons be incorporated into mainstream health plans. While the poor generally would not be able to enroll in higher-cost plans (unless they can afford higher premium payments), they would have access to all plans whose premiums are less than the weighted average premium. Moreover, since premiums payments financed by Medicaid would be merged with those paid by employers, health care plans would receive exactly the same premium (subject to risk adjustments) for Medicaid recipients as they would for other Americans. Thus, in theory, health care plans should be equally interested in low-income and "regular" clients. However, if the risk adjustments are crude and fail to adequately compensate health plans for health risks, the poor—who often have complex, costly health problems—may still be unattractive to competing health care plans. While health plans might still try to avoid or underserve some low-income or Medicaid-type clients, it is reasonable to expect that Medicaid clients' access to mainstream health care will generally improve.

Finally, the growth in health care spending for the poor should be slowed under the Clinton plan. As described above, the proposal relies on two basic cost containment measures—structured competition among health plans to reduce costs and expenditure targets—to stem health care spending. To the extent these measures curtail the growth rate of health care spending, Medicaid expenditure growth would be lower than it would be without reform.

The Cooper/Breaux Proposal

The Managed Competition Act, introduced by Representative Jim Cooper and Senator John Breaux features expansion of health care coverage on a voluntary basis as well as cost containment through managed competition. The managed competition concept is similar to that in the Clinton Plan, although this proposal uses *health plan purchasing cooperatives* (HPPCs) instead of regional health alliances and *accountable health plans* (AHPs) in lieu of health plans. Individuals and firms with less than 100 employees would get AHPs through their HPPC. Medicaid would be abolished and replaced with a program that subsidizes AHP purchases for low-income persons. The proposal requires that AHPs offer open enrollment to all individuals. In addition, AHPs would be banned from denying coverage due to pre-existing health conditions and from using experience rating. AHPs are allowed to require cost-sharing for services, except for preventive care. Large firms may set up their own AHPs to cover their employees. To further contain costs, employers' tax deductions for health insurance will be capped, causing them to be more cost conscious in purchasing insurance.

While employers are required to offer health care coverage, the Cooper/Breaux plan does not require employers to pay for such coverage; premium payment by employers is strictly voluntary. If an employer decides not to pay premiums for its employees, employees are fully responsible for the premium payments if they want health care coverage. Because health insurance would be voluntary, individuals may opt to not purchase insurance; there would be no employer or individual mandates.

The Cooper/Breaux plan calls for repealing existing Medicaid legislation. In its place, a new, federally financed program—covering acute and preventive care—would be established that would pay health care premiums for all persons with incomes below 100 percent of the poverty level. In addition, the new program will provide subsidies, up to some capped amount, on a sliding scale for individuals with incomes between 100 and 200 percent of poverty. As mentioned, the new program would only provide acute and preventive care protection; long-term care is not included in the benefit package. The plan mandates that long-term care for the poor and disabled would eventually become a state responsibility without federal financial participation.

In terms of our four assessment criteria, the Cooper/Breaux bill would extend full coverage, with no cost-sharing for services, to those in poverty. The program provides limited protection for the near poor. Those between 100 and 200 percent of poverty would have to pay for some fraction of their premiums, cost-sharing would be required, and government funds available to subsidize premiums for this population would be capped.

It is difficult to judge the depth of benefits under the Cooper/Breaux plan at present. The proposal states that an independent national health board will establish the standard health benefits package which will include a full range of medical and preventive services. Beyond this, benefit details are limited.

The Cooper/Breaux proposal features several cost control measures. Most prominently, it relies on managed competition among AHPs to control costs. Unlike the Clinton plan, the HPPCs would primarily cover small businesses, so there is a smaller pool of covered persons. This may reduce the competitive pressures for the pricing of insurance plans. If intense price competition develops, the plan should contain costs. However, if price competition does not develop or people are relatively insensitive to price in making decisions about their health care plan, the Cooper/Breaux plan will not be able to control costs. If the latter happens, health care spending for the poor could grow faster than it would otherwise. The Cooper/Breaux plan does not include global budgets to provide additional cost controls, a feature of the Clinton plan. Beyond managed competition, cost containment is also expected from reducing Medicare spending growth through program cutbacks, repealing Medicaid, reforming medical malpractice insurance, and limiting the tax deductibility of health care premiums.

Because the Cooper plan guarantees health care coverage for those in poverty, most of the existing inequities among states' coverage of the poor should be eliminated. For the near poor interstate differences should also be reduced, but not eliminated. There may still be interstate differences due to the voluntary nature of the plan and regional discrepancies in the effective price of subsidized insurance because of regional differences in the price of insurance. Since long-term care will become a state responsibility under the proposal, differences in access to such services will likely increase across states.

The Chafee/Thomas Proposal

The proposal from Senator John Chafee and Representative William Thomas—the Health Equity and Access Reform Today Act—calls for phasing in universal coverage for acute and preventive services.

Beginning in 1997, federal subsidies to buy health insurance for those up to 90 percent of poverty would be available. By the year 2005 the subsidies would extend to 240 percent of poverty and all Americans would have to purchase health insurance. However, the implementation of these provisions depends on whether certain budgetary savings are achieved. If Medicaid and Medicare savings targets are not attained, then the subsidies and individual mandate may be postponed, perhaps indefinitely. The proposal would cap Medicaid spending, phase out Medicaid DSH funding, increase Medicare Part B coinsurance and reduce Medicare spending growth.

Additionally, states would be required to establish purchasing cooperatives for firms with 100 or fewer employees and individuals. The purchasing cooperatives will oversee the offering of qualified health plans to individuals and employers. Again, the concept of managed competition is a critical component of the plan. A relatively broad standard benefit package will be provided, with benefits to be determined later.

The plan would also obtain revenues from treating as taxable income any employer contributions to health insurance that exceed certain limits. By reducing the tax deductibility of health insurance, employer's cost consciousness should also be heightened.

Similar to the preceding proposal, the Chafee/Thomas plan only requires that individuals and employees in firms with fewer than 100 workers would be in the health care purchasing cooperatives and does not include global budgeting. Although this plan features strong cost-containment policies for Medicare and Medicaid, the likelihood of successfully controlling costs in the private market is more limited.

The Chafee/Thomas plan retains Medicaid, although it would gradually permit states to enroll Medicaid clients into the qualified health plans in lieu of the regular Medicaid programs. At first, up to 15 percent of AFDC and SSI clients could join the qualified health plans, although the percentage increases over time. If, however, qualified health plan costs are higher than standard Medicaid payment rates, states will have a disincentive to place Medicaid clients in the private health insurance pools. If Medicaid is kept separate and is subject to stringent growth targets, it is likely that Medicaid beneficiaries not enrolled in qualified health plans will have less access to health providers than the general populace.

The proposal would cap federal Medicaid payments for acute and preventive care (on a per capita basis) and eliminate DSH payments. The federal caps would be based on historical spending trends and states would be at risk for further costs. For beneficiaries who remain in Medicaid and for long-term care recipients, interstate differences may actually be exacerbated because of the increased pressure on state budgets. However, for other low income persons (who would be eligible for the federal subsidies for the low-income) there would be significant reductions in interstate differences in access.

The Wellstone/McDermott Proposal

The proposal of Senator Paul Wellstone and Representative James McDermott is a single-payer plan that would be federally controlled, but administered by each state. All individuals would be enrolled in the same system, regardless of income or employment. The Medicaid and Medicare programs would fully merge with the new systems.

The proposal calls for a broad and comprehensive benefit package, including acute, preventive and long-term care benefits. Individuals would pay neither premiums nor copayments for acute and preventive medical services. Those over 65 years of age would be required to pay premiums for long-term care insurance, although subsidies will be available for the low-income elderly. The bill would establish a broad system of long-term care, including home and community-based services.

Financing would be through a combination of new taxes, redirection of state and federal funds and premiums for long-term care. New taxes would include "sin" taxes, such as increases in cigarette taxes, and payroll taxes. States would be required to contribute 15 percent of the costs, although it is not clear how this contribution would be distributed across states.

Although federal taxes would be increased substantially by this plan, it would eliminate most private costs of health care currently paid by employers and individuals. Through the virtual elimination of private insurance plans and creation of uniform state systems, there is the potential for dramatic reductions in administrative costs of the health care system. The Congressional Budget Office estimated that a single-payer plan could be most effective in reducing overall national health care costs, although it increases federal costs substantially.

The Wellstone/McDermott plan would give federal and state governments broad power to establish and enforce strict cost controls. The proposal would establish annual global budgets for health care and limit the growth in spending to increases in gross domestic product. States would control health care spending by limiting physician fees and hospital and nursing home budgets, and negotiating prescription drug prices with drug companies.

Although many are concerned about the substantial increases in governmental costs and power over the health care system that are associated with a single-payer plan, from the perspective of the poor, it clearly meets each of our criteria. All of the poor and near poor would be covered. Moreover, the benefit package is broad and requires no cost-sharing for acute and preventive services. There would be no differences in access to benefits across states. Medicaid beneficiaries as well as all of the remaining poor and near poor would be covered in the same way as all other Americans. The costs of serving the poor would be kept under control through the global budgets. In addition, any efforts to control costs through constraining hospital or physician spending would presumably affect poor and rich alike.

The Michel Proposal

The proposal by Representative Robert Michel calls for incremental improvements in the health care system. It would expand Medicaid coverage, deal with some problems in the insurance market, and otherwise features little structural changes in the existing health care system. Although it would provide some useful reforms to the health insurance marketplace, such as creation of voluntary insurance purchase cooperatives, limitation of pre-existing condition exclusions, and standardization of some insurance marketing practices, it would not offer universal coverage nor does it feature strong cost containment mechanisms.

The Michel plan would restructure Medicaid and permits expansion. States would be allowed to create state health allowance plans that subsidize Medicaid clients' enrollment into private health insurance plans that are at least equal in actuarial value to their Medicaid benefits. Medicaid clients can elect to join the health allowance plan in lieu of Medicaid. States would be required to cover persons up to 100 percent of poverty, unless this would increase state costs to a higher level than they would otherwise spend. So, if expansion of the state health allowance program causes states' costs to increase, they can lower the income standard below 100 percent of poverty. States may also expand state health allowance eligibility up to 200 percent of poverty with sliding-scale contributions from beneficiaries. Since Medicaid payment rates are usually much lower than private insurance, it is difficult to conceive of circumstances in which the state health allowance plans could be cheaper than current Medicaid benefits, so it seems unlikely that the 100 percent of poverty eligibility standard could apply very often.

In terms of our criteria, the Michel plan might expand Medicaid eligibility for some low-income individuals, although this would largely be at states' discretion. In addition, the insurance reforms might help reduce the cost of private insurance for a limited number of low-income persons. But, in general, the Michel plan would not substantially expand coverage for the low-income.

Concerning differences in access between states, these would remain and could, in fact, be exacerbated if the Michel proposal were adopted. The state health allowance programs might permit some Medicaid clients into private insurance plans, but it is not clear with what frequency this would occur given the budget-neutrality protections built into the plan. The differences in access between Medicaid and private insurance clients would probably not change very much. Because the Michel plan has no real cost containment provisions, Medicaid expenditures would probably grow over time.

Summary

Each of the major health reform proposals that have been introduced in Congress would solve at least some of the problems with the current Medicaid program and with health insurance for the poor. Under even the most limited plan, that of Representative Michel, health insurance coverage for those under poverty would increase somewhat. The Clinton and Wellstone/McDermott plans have the strongest guarantees of universal coverage, although the Chafee/Thomas proposal aims toward universal coverage and the Cooper/Breaux plan would provide assistance to those under 200 percent of poverty.

But the value of the insurance coverage would differ substantially among proposals. Some offer extensive benefit packages, while the range of services is unclear in others. Although the Clinton and Wellstone/McDermott plans would expand long-term care, the other plans have no long-term care programs and would leave these responsibilities to the current Medicaid program or to states.

Proposals that retain separate Medicaid programs (Michel and Chafee/Thomas) may hold down governmental costs, but low payment rates and stigma associated with Medicaid could still impair the willingness of physicians and other health care providers to treat Medicaid patients. The Clinton and Cooper/Breaux proposals would mainstream Medicaid acute and preventive services into private health insurance plans. However, since the governmental subsidies would be limited to low-cost plans, it seems likely that low-income clients would enroll in strict managed care plans, such as closed panel HMOs. Though the quality of services might be similar, they would have somewhat less choice about health care than middle class patients. The Wellstone/McDermott plan, by contrast, would provide more uniform access for people, regardless of income.

The cost of serving the poor also varies across plans. Those with stronger general cost containment provisions, such as the Clinton or Wellstone/McDermott proposals, are probably more likely to serve the poor at a lower cost. The two that rely most on managed competition (Chafee/Thomas and Cooper/Breaux) may also bring costs under control successfully, but evidence on the effectiveness of managed competition is less clear.

A reasonable criterion for national health reform is the degree to which it is truly national and treats people similarly across states. As discussed above, there are important differences from the perspective of the low-income beneficiaries.

Although the past decade witnessed tremendous growth and change in Medicaid, it is clear that national and state health reform proposals now under discussion (and sometimes already implemented by states) could bring about even more radical changes. Although Medicaid's ability to serve the poor grew and interstate disparities shrank over the past decade, it seems clear that policymakers are calling for even greater change. But the past decade's changes in Medicaid should not be dismissed summarily. Without the past decade's growth in Medicaid participation and expenditures, the additional costs of providing universal health insurance would be even more expensive and less politically viable. Even parts of Medicaid that caused the greatest ire, such as disproportionate-share programs, are now important budgetary building blocks in a grander foundation of health care reform. In grappling with the massive and complex problems of health care reform, the nation faces one of the greatest public policy challenges of recent times. While it is still too early to know the outcome of these debates, it is self-evident that the structure and financing of health care for low-income, disabled and aged Americans will continue to be a major focus of public policy in the future.

APPENDIX A: THE MEDICAID PRICE INDEX

As noted in the text, the price index we employed to adjust for changes in spending is an update of previous indices described in Holahan and Cohen (1986). The HCFA market basket indices and MC-CPI components used to create the Medicaid price index (MPI) and its components were as follows:

Acute Care
Inpatient hospital	HCFA hospital market basket
Physician, laboratory, X-ray	MC-CPI physician services component
Outpatient hospital	HCFA hospital market basket
Prescription drugs	MC-CPI prescription drugs component
Other services	MC-CPI medical care component

Long-term Care
Home health	HCFA home health market basket
Nursing home	HCFA nursing home market basket
ICF/MR	HCFA nursing home market basket
Inpatient mental care	HCFA nursing home market basket

The index for total services is a composite of price indices for services (as just outlined) purchased by Medicaid programs, weighted by the relative importance of those services. Weights were based on the proportion of total expenditures accounted for by each service. For example, if inpatient hospital expenditures accounted for 25 percent of total expenditures, price changes in the HCFA hospital market basket index were weighted to account for 25 percent of the change in the index used to adjust total expenditures for inflation. The weighted-adjusted price indexes for each service were then summed to produce a weighted average index. The index, therefore, reflects the real cost of services purchased by the Medicaid program, based on equivalent prices for the general health care sector.

To create the indices for acute and long-term care services, price changes for the appropriate service components (as outlined here) were weighted and then summed to produce a weighted average index for each service group, that is, long-term care and acute care services, separately. Total service indices were calculated separately for each eligibility group. For example, the index for children is a composite of the price indices for services purchased by children, weighted by the relative importance of the services in a manner similar to that just described.

The values in table 2.6, the percentage of total expenditure growth between 1988 and 1992 due to each factor, were calculated as shares of total expenditure growth during that period. Total expenditure growth is the product of recipient growth, utilization, and excess reimbursement (real expenditures per recipient) and medical price inflation, as represented in the following equation:

$$\Delta X = \Delta \frac{X'}{N} \times \Delta N \times i_{Med}, \tag{B.1}$$

where X is expenditures, X' is real expenditures, N is recipients, and i_{Med} is medical price inflation. In logarithmic form the relationship is:

$$\ln\left(\frac{X_{92}}{X_{88}}\right) = \ln\left(\frac{\dfrac{X_{92}}{N_{92} \times i_{Med}}}{\dfrac{X_{88}}{N_{88}}}\right) + \ln\left(\frac{N_{92}}{N_{88}}\right) + \ln(i_{Med}), \tag{B.2}$$

from which the shares of growth can be easily calculated by dividing each of the three elements on the right-hand side of the equation by the left-hand side of the equation.

The formula to derive the share of total expenditure growth due to increased utilization and excess reimbursement is:

$$S_{u+er} = \frac{\ln\left(\dfrac{\dfrac{X_{92}}{N_{92} \times i_{Med}}}{\dfrac{X_{88}}{N_{88}}}\right)}{\ln\left(\dfrac{X_{92}}{X_{88}}\right)}. \tag{B.3}$$

Similarly, the formulas to calculate the share of total expenditure growth due to enrollment growth and inflation are:

$$S_{enr} = \frac{\ln\left(\dfrac{N_{92}}{N_{88}}\right)}{\ln\left(\dfrac{X_{92}}{X_{88}}\right)}, \; S_{mpi} = \frac{\ln(i_{Med})}{\ln\left(\dfrac{X_{92}}{X_{88}}\right)}. \tag{B.4}$$

These shares of expenditure growth were calculated for spending on each type of service for each recipient group. In these calculations, total expenditures exclude spending on Medicare, health maintenance organizations (HMOs), and group health payments. However, for presentation in table 2.6, these shares are adjusted to represent the share of total expenditures with Medicare, HMOs, and group health payments included.

In table 2.7, these shares are adjusted again to first represent the share of total expenditures with all growth factors included in table 2.6 plus disproportionate-share payments. Also in table 2.7, we show the share of total spending with all growth factors plus disproportionate-share payments net of revenues obtained from special financing programs—provider tax and donation programs and intergovernmental transfer programs.

REFERENCES

American Hospital Association. 1992. "Unsponsored Hospital Care and Medicaid Shortfalls, 1980–91: A Fact Sheet Update." Chicago: Author, November (rev.).

American Medical Association. 1991. "Physician Participation in Medicaid." *Physician Marketplace Update*, July.

Anderson, G., and W. Scanlon. 1993. "Medicaid Payment Policy and the Boren Amendment." In *Medicaid Financing Crisis: Balancing Responsibilities, Priorities and Dollars*, edited by D. Rowland, J. Feder, and A. Salganicoff (82–94). American Association for the Advancement of Science.

Bachman, S., D. Beatrice, and S. Altman. 1987. "Implementing Change: Lessons for Medicaid Reformers." *Journal of Health Politics, Policy and Law* 12(2): 237–51.

Barancik, S., and I. Shapiro. 1992. *Where Have All the Dollars Gone? A State by State Analysis of Income Disparities over the 1980s*. Washington, D.C.: Center on Budget and Policy Priorities.

Burner, S. T., D. R. Waldo, and D. R. McKusick. 1992. "National Health Expenditures Projections through 2930." *Health Care Financing Review* 14(1): 1–30.

Burwell, B. 1993. "State Responses to Medicaid to Medicaid Estate Planning." Systemetrics, Cambridge, Ma., May.

Chang, D., and J. Holahan. 1990. *Medicaid Spending in the 1980s: The Access-Cost Containment Trade-Off Revisited*. Washington, D.C.: Urban Institute Press.

Cohen, J. 1989. "Medicaid Policy and the Substitution of Hospital Outpatient Care for Physician Care." *Health Services Research* 24: 33–66.

Committee on Ways and Means. See U.S. Congress. House. Committee on Ways and Means.

Congressional Budget Office. 1992a. "Factors Contributing to the Growth of the Medicaid Program." Staff Memorandum. Washington, D.C.: Author, May.

———. 1992b. "Projections of National Health Expenditures." Washington, D.C.: Author, October.

————. 1993. "Responses to Uncompensated Care and Public-Program Controls on Spending: Do Hospitals Cost Shift?" Washington, D.C.: Author, May.

Congressional Research Service. 1988. *Medicaid Source Book: Background Data and Analysis*. Subcommittee on Health and the Environment, U.S. House of Representatives. 100th Congress, 2d Session. Committee Print 100-AA, November.

————. 1992. "Medicaid: Recent Trends in Beneficiaries and Spending." Report for Congress. Washington, D.C.: Author, March 27.

————. 1993. *Medicaid Source Book: Background Data and Analysis, A 1993 Update*. Subcommittee on Health and the Environment, U.S. House of Representatives. 103rd Congress, 1st Session. Committee Print 103-A, U.S. Government Printing Office, Washington, D.C., January.

Connell, F. A. 1992. "Access and Outcomes in Washington's First Steps Project." Paper presented at the Fourteenth Annual Research Conference of the Association for Public Policy Analysis and Management, Denver, October.

Davis, K., and C. Schoen. 1978. *Health and the War on Poverty: A Ten-Year Appraisal*. Washington, D.C.: Brookings Institution.

Dubay, L., G. Kenney, S. Norton, and B. Cohen. 1993. "Local Responses to Medicaid Expansions for Pregnant Women." Urban Institute Working Paper 6217-02. Washington, D.C.: Urban Institute, March.

Erdman, K., and S. Wolfe. 1987. *Poor Health Care for Poor Americans: A Ranking of State Medicaid Programs*. Washington, D.C.: Public Citizen Health Research Group.

Families USA. 1993. *The Medicare Buy-In: A Promise Unfilled*. Washington, D.C.: The Families USA Foundation, March.

Feder, J., D. Rowland, J. Holahan, A. Salganicoff, and D. Heslam. 1993. "The Medicaid Cost Explosion: Cause and Consequences." Menlo Park, Calif.: Kaiser Commission on the Future of Medicaid.

Federal Register, The. 1993. "Medicaid Program: Limitations on Aggregate Payments to Disproportionate Share Hospitals, Federal Fiscal Year 1993," Vol. 58, p. 43184.

Gold, R. B., A. Kenney, and S. Singh. 1987. "Blessed Events and the Bottom Line: Financing Maternity Care in the United States." New York: Alan Guttmacher Institute.

Gold, S. 1993. "The State Budget Context: How Medicaid Fits In." In *Medicaid Financing Crisis: Balancing Responsibilities, Priorities and Dollars*, edited by D. Rowland, J. Feder, and A. Salganicoff (133–54). Washington, D.C.: American Association for the Advancement of Science.

Health Insurance Association of America. 1992. *Source Book of Health Insurance Data—1992*. Washington, D.C.: Author.

Health Policy Alternatives. 1992. *Medicaid Provider Tax and Donation Issues*. Washington, D.C.: Author, July.

Holahan, J. 1988. "The Impact of Alternative Hospital Payment Systems on Medicaid Costs." *Inquiry*, 25(4): 517–32.

Holahan, J. 1991. "Medicaid Physician Fees, 1990: The Results of a New Survey." Urban Institute Working Paper No. 6110-01. Washington, D.C.: Urban Institute.

Holahan, J., and J. Cohen. 1986. *Medicaid: The Trade-Off between Cost Containment and Access to Care.* Washington, D.C.: Urban Institute Press.

Holahan, J., T. A. Coughlin, L. Ku, D. Heslam, and C. Winterbottom. 1992. "The States' Response to Medicaid Financing Crises: Case Studies Report." Baltimore, Md.: Kaiser Commission on the Future of Medicaid, December.

Hurley, R., D. Freund, and J. Paul. 1993. *Managed Care in Medicaid.* Ann Arbor, Mich.: Health Administration Press.

Intergovernmental Health Policy Project. 1989. *State Systems for Hospital Payment.* Washington, D.C.: Author, April.

————. 1993a. *Profile of the States and Health Care Reform.* Report prepared for the Henry J. Kaiser Family Foundation, Washington, D.C., July.

————. 1993b. *State Health Notes* 14(147): 7.

————. 1993c. *State Health Notes* 14(157): 1–2,8.

Johns, L. 1989. "Selective Contracting in California: An Update." *Health Affairs* 26(3): 345–53.

Kosterlitz, J. 1992. "Managing Medicaid." *National Journal,* May 9: 1111–15.

Kronick, R. 1991. "Health Insurance, 1979–1989: The Frayed Connection between Employment and Insurance." *Inquiry* 28: 318–22.

Ku, L., M. Ellwood, and J. Klemm. 1990. "Deciphering Medicaid Data: Issues and Needs." *Health Care Financing Review* (annual suppl.): 35–46.

Lakin, K. C., T. M. Jaskulski, B. K. Hill, et al. 1989. "Medicaid Services for Persons with Mental Retardation and Related Conditions." University of Minnesota, Institute on Community Integration. Minneapolis, Minn.

Lakin, K. C., and M. J. Hall. 1990. "Medicaid-financed Residential Care for Persons with Mental Retardation." *Health Care Financing Review* (annual suppl.): 149–60.

Lakin, K. C., R. W. Prouty, C. C. White, et al. 1990. Intermediate Care Facilities for Persons with Mental Retardation (ICF-MRs). Program Utilization and Resident Characteristics Report 31. University of Minnesota, Institute on Community Integration. Minneapolis, Minn.

LaPlante, M. 1993. "State Estimates of Disability in America." In *Disability Statistics Report,* U.S. National Institute on Disability and Rehabilitation Research, U.S. Department of Education. Washington, D.C.: U.S. Government Printing Office.

Lav, I., E. Lazere, R. Greenstein, and S. Gold. 1993. *The States and the Poor: How Budget Decisions Affected Low Income People in 1992.* Washington, D.C.: Center on Budget and Policy Priorities, February.

Levit, K. R., G. L. Olin, and S. W. Letsch. 1992. "American's Health Insurance Coverage, 1980–91." *Health Care Financing Review* 14(1): 31–57.

Lewis-Idema, D., M. Falik, T. Ricketts, J. Kolimags, and G. Wright. 1992. "Effects of Increased FQHC Revenue on Community Health Centers." Report to the Health Resources and Services Administration from Mathematica Policy Research (with MDS Associates and the Cecil C. Sheps Center for Health Services Research, University of North Carolina). (photocopy).

McConnell, S. 1991. "The Increase in Food Stamp Program Participation between 1989 and 1990." Washington, D.C.: Mathematica Policy Research, August.

Miller, M., and Gengler, D. Forthcoming. "Primary Care Case Management and Medicaid Utilization." *Health Care Financing Review.*

Miller, V. 1992. "Medicaid Financing Mechanisms and Federal Limits: A State Perspective." In *Medicaid Provider Taxes and Donation Issues.* Washington, D.C.: Health Policy Alternatives, July.

Moon, M. 1993. *Medicare Now and in the Future.* Washington, D.C.: Urban Institute Press.

Morgan, D. 1993. "Medicaid Windfall Cuts N.H. Deficit." *Washington Post,* Feb. 28.

National Association of Public Hospitals. 1989. "Revised State Medicaid Policies for Disproportionate Share Hospitals: A Status Report." Washington, D.C.: Author, May.

————. 1991. "Revised State Medicaid Policies for Disproportionate Share Hospitals: An Updated Status Report." Washington, D.C.: Author.

NASBO. *See* National Association of State Budget Officers.

National Association of State Budget Officers. 1993a. "Balancing the State Medicaid Budget, FY 1992 and FY 1993." Washington, D.C.: Author.

————. 1993b. *1992 State Expenditure Report.* Washington, D.C.: Author.

National Governors Association. 1989. *Medicaid Payment for Nursing Homes: Skilled Nursing Facilities and Intermediate Care Facilities (1986–89).* Washington, D.C.: Author.

National Governors Association and National Association of State Budget Officers. 1992. *The Fiscal Survey of States.* Washington, D.C.: Author.

Office of the Inspector General, U.S. Department of Health and Human Services. 1992. "Use of Emergency Rooms by Medicaid Recipients." OEI-06-90-00180. Washington, D.C.: Author.

Office of Management and Budget. 1991. Better Management for Better Medicaid Estimates. Washington, D.C.: Author, July.

Piper, J. M., E. F. Mitchel, and W. A. Ray. 1992. "Expanded Medicaid Coverage for Pregnant Women to 100 Percent of the Federal Poverty Line." Paper presented at the Fourteenth Annual Research Conference of the Association for Public Policy Analysis and Management, Denver, October.

Reilly, T. W., S. B. Clauser, and D. K. Baugh. 1990. "Trends in Medicaid Payments and Utilization." *Health Care Financing Review* (annual suppl.): 15–33.

Reinhardt, U. 1985. "20 Years of Medicare and Medicaid: Symposium." *Health Care Financing Review* (annual suppl.): 105–11.

Rogal, D. L., and W. D. Helms. 1993. "State Models: Tracking States' Efforts to Reform Their Health System." *Health Affairs* 12(2): 27–31.

Rosenbaum, S. 1993. "Medicaid Expansion and Access to Care." In *Medicaid Financing Crisis: Balancing Responsibilities, Priorities and Dollars,* edited by D. Rowland, J. Feder, and A. Salganicoff. Washington, D.C.: American Association for the Advancement of Science.

Sullivan v. Zebley. 493 U.S. 521 (1990).

U.S. Bureau of the Census. 1992. *Poverty in the United States: 1991.* Current Population Reports, ser. P-60, no. 181. Washington, D.C.: U.S. Government Printing Office.

U.S. Congress. House. Committee on Ways and Means. 1993. *Overview of Entitlement Programs: 1992 Green Book.* Washington, D.C.: U.S. Government Printing Office.

U.S. General Accounting Office. 1991. "Prenatal Care: Early Success in Enrolling Women Made Eligible by Medicaid Expansions." GAO/PEMD 91-10. Washington, D.C.: Author, February.

————. 1993. "Medicaid: States Turn to Managed Care to Improve Access and Control Costs." GAO/HRD-93-46. Washington, D.C.: Author, March.

Wade, M. 1993. "Medicaid Managed Care: The Effects of Fee-for-Service Case Management on Enrollees' Service Use." Urban Institute Working Paper 6317-01. Washington, D.C.: Urban Institute, May.

Welch, W. P. 1992. "Alternative Geographic Adjustments in Medicare Payment to Health Maintenance Organizations." *Health Care Financing Review* 13(3): 97–110.

Welch, W. P., S. Katz, and S. Zuckerman. 1992. "Physician Fee Levels: Medicare versus Canada." Urban Institute Working Paper 6185-02. Washington, D.C.: Urban Institute, Sept.

Wilder v. Virginia Hospital Association. 110 S.Ct. 2510 (1990).

Winterbottom, C. 1993. "Trends in Health Insurance Coverage: 1988–1991." Urban Institute Working Paper. Washington, D.C.: Urban Institute, June.

Wolfe, B., and R. Haveman. 1990. "Trends in the Prevalence of Work Disability from 1962 to 1984 and Their Correlates." *Milbank Quarterly* 68(1): 53–80.

ABOUT THE AUTHORS

Teresa A. Coughlin is currently a senior research associate with the Health Policy Center of the Urban Institute. She has conducted research on a variety of health care issues, with a special focus on long-term care and policy for low-income persons. Prior to coming to the Institute she was a research fellow at the Agency for Health Care Policy and Research, where she was engaged in research on various aspects of long-term care.

Leighton Ku is a senior research associate in the Urban Institute's Health Policy Center. In addition to his research on Medicaid, he has examined the areas of maternal and child health, AIDS prevention, family planning, and nutrition assistance. Beyond his work at the Institute, he is also an associate professorial lecturer in public policy at the George Washington University. Prior to his association with the Urban Institute, he was a research manager at SysteMetrics, a Pew Health Policy Fellow at Boston University, and a policy analyst at the Food and Nutrition Service, USDA.

John Holahan is the director of the Institute's Health Policy Center. He has written extensively on a range of health care issues, including Medicaid and the uninsured, physician payment, hospital cost containment, and nursing home reimbursement. His current work focuses on health care reform and financing. Recent books of his published by the Urban Institute Press include: *Balancing Access, Costs, and Politics: The American Context for Health System Reform* (1991), with Marilyn Moon, W. Pete Welch, and Stephen Zuckerman; *Medicaid Spending in the 1980s: The Access-Cost Containment Trade-off Revisited*, with Deborah Chang (1990); and *Medicaid: The Trade-off between Cost Containment and Access to Care*, with Joel Cohen (1986).